Tendinitis:
its etiology
and treatment

Tendinitis: its etiology and treatment

Sandra Curwin, B.Sc.PT, M.Sc.
William D. Stanish, M.D., F.R.C.S.

The Collamore Press
D.C. Heath and Company
LEXINGTON, MASSACHUSETTS
TORONTO

Published simultaneously in Canada

Printed in the United States of America

International Standard Book Number: 0-669-07394-6

Library of Congress Catalog Card Number: 83-72496

Design by Outside Designs

Library of Congress Cataloging in Publication Data
Curwin, Sandra.
    Tendinitis: its etiology and treatment.

    Bibliography: p.
    Includes index.
    1. Tendinitis. I. Stanish, William D. II. Title.
[DNLM: 1. Tendinitis—Etiology. 2. Tendinitis—Therapy.
WE 600 C982t]
RC935.T4C87 1984   616.7′5   83-72496
ISBN 0-669-07394-6

Contents

Introduction

This book is about tendinitis, that annoying soft-tissue lesion that can be so difficult to deal with because so many times it simply will not go away. This is naturally quite frustrating for all concerned: athlete, doctor, physiotherapist, coach. The list may become even longer if the problem remains unsolved.

What is tendinitis? Literally, tendinitis is inflammation of a tendon. Since some sort of tendon is associated with each of the body's approximately 640 muscles, there are many potential sites for injury. In this book we focus on those sites that are most common—those that occur in runners (Achilles tendinitis), jumpers (jumper's knee), and racquet players (tennis elbow).

Defining tendinitis does not bring us any closer to understanding its true nature, or its pathogenesis and treatment. These questions have plagued clinicians for many years. The result is a vast assortment of suggested remedies, from rest, immobilization, or even surgery to resisted exercise.

Our approach to tendinitis is based on the theory that the tensile strength of the tendon is inadequate to enable it to meet the demands of athletes and that successful resolution of symptoms will occur only when this situation is remedied. Furthermore, we believe, as did Wolff in 1892, that exercise strengthens and inactivity wastes. This led to the development of the program we currently use to treat tendinitis, which is really the brainchild of Dr. Howard Lamb (who was a medical student when he developed the program, albeit one with a good knowledge of biomechanics).

Before we outline the treatment program and its application to the various types of tendinitis, the structure and function of tendon are reviewed and the pathologic changes that accompany tendinitis are discussed in Chapters 1 and 2. Attention is focused on the mechanical behavior of the tendon during activities and the factors that influence this behavior. The reader should bear in mind that much of this work is theoretical, there being little in the way of direct experimentation on human tendon.

In Chapters 4, 5, and 6, the application of the program to Achilles tendinitis, jumper's knee, and tennis elbow is presented. These chapters also include descriptions of the signs and symptoms of these disorders and tips for differential diagnosis. Finally, in Chapter 8, the results of a survey of the treatment of 200 patients are presented. These results clearly indicate our success with the eccentric exercise program and our frustration with traditional conservative treatment methods.

Tendinitis:
its etiology
and treatment

1. Normal tendon

This chapter deals with the normal tendon and its structure and function. Since tendon's structure determines its response to the tasks imposed on it during activity, this topic is important. Both the ultrastructure of the tendon and other structural factors such as length and cross-sectional area affect the way tendons behave when forces are applied to them; blood supply and metabolic activity affect the rate of healing after injury. Since all these things influence the clinical course of tendinitis, the purpose of this chapter is to lay the groundwork for later discussion of tendinitis and its treatment.

The muscle-tendon unit

Tendons are ropelike structures that connect muscles to bone. The muscles are the prime movers of the body—they contract and produce force. Tendons allow precise application of this force to the limb being moved. Thus we speak of the *muscle-tendon unit*, or a muscle and its attached tendon(s).

Muscles vary widely in size, shape, and complexity (Fig. 1-1). Some are broad and flat with wide, short tendons, such as the gluteus maximus or rectus abdominis. Others such as the fusiform biceps have smaller, rounded, cordlike tendons. The important point here is that while muscle and tendon are structurally separate, functionally they are one unit—the muscle-tendon unit. Thus it is somewhat unrealistic to consider and discuss tendon in isolation from its accompanying muscle, and we encourage the reader to always bear this in mind throughout the following pages.

Structure

The composition and properties of tendon are very similar to those of other soft tissues such as ligaments, joint capsule, interosseous

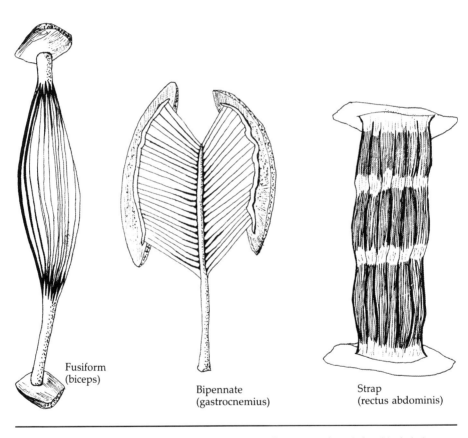

Fusiform
(biceps)

Bipennate
(gastrocnemius)

Strap
(rectus abdominis)

Figure 1-1. The appearance of three different types of muscle found in the body.

membranes, and fascia, all of which supply tensile strength combined with flexibility. The difference lies in the fact that all these structures, except fascia, connect bone to bone, while tendon is interspersed between muscle and bone.

The insertion of tendon into bone involves a gradual transition from tendon to fibrocartilage to mineralized fibrocartilage to lamellar bone. The presence of the fibrocartilage means very few blood vessels traverse the bone-tendon junction. The junction between muscle and tendon is via projections of the tendon fibrils into the muscle membrane at the ends of the fasciculi (Viidik 1973).

Ultrastructure   Tendon is composed of collagen and elastin, two proteins, embedded in a proteoglycan-water matrix or gel. The usual distribution is approximately 2 percent elastin, 30 percent collagen, and 58 to 70 percent water. Collagen accounts for 70 percent of the dry weight of tendon and so is considered the major structural component. All the above substances are produced by cells called *fibroblasts* that are found throughout the tendon and that become more numerous when new connective tissue must be produced, such as during development or in injury repair.

Collagen synthesis parallels that of other protein molecules. Amino acids are assembled into chains that fold into a triple helix (procollagen). As the triple helices leave the cell, enzymes in the extracellular environment remove part of the procollagen molecule; then it is known as *tropocollagen*. The tropocollagen molecule is considered the most fundamental unit in collagenous structures.

Present knowledge suggests that five tropocollagen units join to form a larger fibrous entity, the microfibril. The molecules are assembled in a staggered fashion, with each overlapping its neighbors by about one-quarter of its length (Fig. 1-2).

---

1. Normal tendon

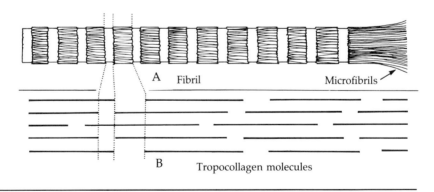

Figure 1-2. *The staggering of tropocollagen molecules to form microfibrils and fibrils.*

Next the microfibrils group into subfibrils, which in turn form fibrils—the basic load-bearing units of ligaments or tendons. The collagen fibrils appear cross-striated, or banded, under the electron microscope because of the staggering of the tropocollagen molecules and gaps in the head-to-tail arrangement of the molecules.

Groups of parallel fibrils, surrounded by the matrix, are known as *fibers.* These may be as long as the tendon itself, and they associate into larger groups (primary tendon bundles) which then aggregate into fascicles. Surrounding the fascicles is a sheath, the endotenon, through which nerves and blood vessels run. These fascicles are the smallest collagenous structures that can be mechanically tested (Butler et al. 1978). Fibroblasts are found inside the fascicles between the primary fiber bundles. Groups of fascicles, surrounded by a second sheath called the epitenon, form the tendon proper. Outside the epitenon is a third sheath, the paratenon. Small amounts of fluid between the epitenon and paratenon provide lubrication, preventing friction and damage to the tendon.

This complicated structure has been best described by Kastelic, Galeski, and Baer (1978) who termed it the "hierarchical organization of tendon" (Fig. 1-3). The fibers and primary fiber bundles were not described by these authors, although they have been by others, which reflects the lack of agreement about tendon's structure. The fibers and primary fiber bundles may be considered to reside between the fibril and fascicle level.

The collagen fibrils, though they are arranged longitudinally, are not straight; they appear zigzagged, or crimped (Fig. 1-4). This may be due to transverse mechanical interaction between fibrils or to

1. Normal tendon

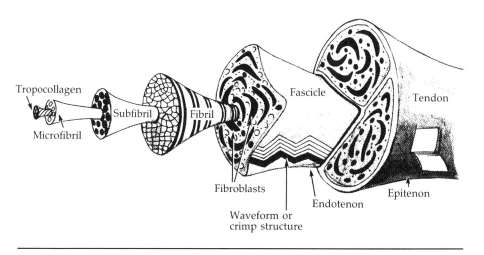

Figure 1-3. The hierarchical organization of the tendon, showing the various stages from molecule to tendon. Redrawn with permission from Kastelic, J., Galeski, A., Baer, E., The multicomposite structure of tendon. Connect. Tissue Res. 6:11–23, *1978.*

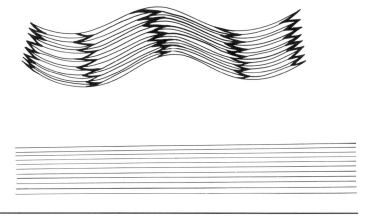

Figure 1-4. The collagen fibrils appear wavy when relaxed, but lose this crimped appearance when stretched.

buckling caused by shrinking of the interfibrillar matrix with age. This wavy configuration, a characteristic feature of tendon, disappears when the tendon is stretched.

Mechanics and function

Tendon's mechanical behavior depends on its structure, as previously described. Its function is to transmit forces from muscle to bone. Since muscle produces force only when it is contracting, this has a stretching effect on the tendon, known in mechanical circles as a tensile force. Other types of forces, such as compressive and shear, also may be applied to soft tissues (Fig. 1-5).

Tendon withstands tensile forces well, resists shear forces less well, and provides little resistance to compressive forces. Bone, however, withstands compression much better than tension. Tendons must be flexible to allow unhindered movement and redirection of force "around corners." For example, the extensor pollicis longus passes around the radial tubercle, runs underneath the extensor retinaculum, and inserts finally on the distal phalanx of the thumb (Fig. 1-6). Note that the tendon is surrounded by a synovial sheath that reduces friction, a common feature in cases where tendons must pass beneath restricting structures.

The tensile force applied to the tendon is resisted mainly by the collagen, which is characterized by poor elasticity but great mechanical strength. Because the collagen fibrils are crimped, the initial response to tensile force is straightening of the fibers so that these waves, or crimps, disappear. Greater loads stress the fibrils themselves. The typical response of tendon to applied tensile force is shown in Figure 1-7.

---

1. Normal tendon

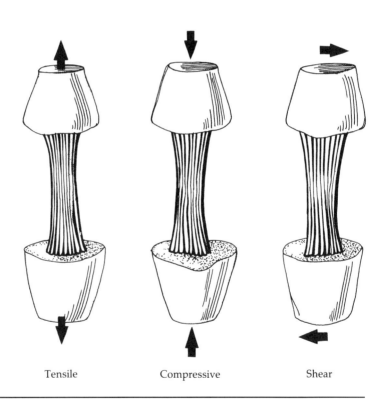

Tensile   Compressive   Shear

Figure 1-5. Types of force to which tendon may be subjected.

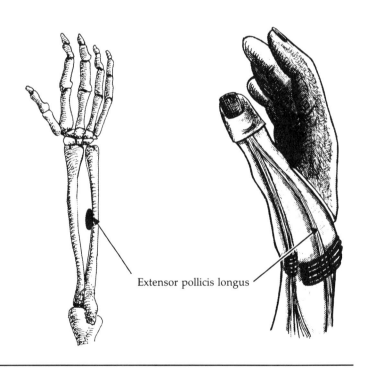

Figure 1-6. Extensor pollicis longus, illustrating the curved paths that muscle-tendon units sometimes follow between origin and insertion.

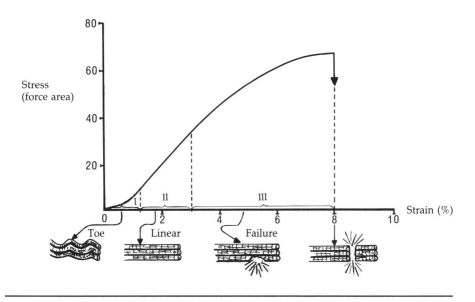

Figure 1-7. A typical stress-strain curve for tendon.

The initial, concave portion of the curve (region I) is called the *toe* region. Under the conditions represented by this part of the curve, little force is required to elongate the tissue, since the fibrils are straightening. This portion of the curve is felt to be governed by shearing within the matrix. As more force is applied, the fibrils straighten and the force-time curve becomes linear, which means that greater magnitudes of force are necessary to elongate the tendon. As more force is applied, some fibers begin to fail (in region III). This, of course, increases the load on those fibers that remain intact, and more and more fibers rupture. As this happens, the tendon bears less load, although it may or may not be completely ruptured at this point.

Size

The same is true for both muscle and tendon: The more fibers present, or the larger those fibers, the more force the tendon can withstand. Thus there is a direct correlation between cross-sectional area and applied load (Fig. 1-8).

Increased size means, in effect, that the tendon is more resistant to stretch, that it is stiffer. Since less elongation accompanies the increase in force, the fibers deform less.

Another physical factor that can influence the tendon's response to tensile force is its length. Longer fibers mean greater elongation at the same load (Fig. 1-9). Thus the ideal situation is long fibers and lots of them.

Because tendon's mechanical behavior depends on its physical size, force-elongation curves must be adjusted to remove the effects of these physical parameters before comparisons can be made between tissue from different tendons. Dividing the force by the cross-sectional area yields the force per unit area, known as *stress;* dividing the change in length by the original length determines the relative

---

1. *Normal tendon*

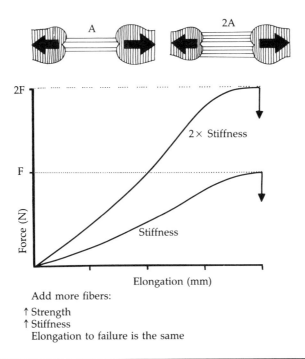

Figure 1-8. The effect of area on tendon behavior. Note that the larger tendon is "stiffer"; that is, more force is borne per unit of elongation. Redrawn with permission from Butler, D.L., Grood, E.S., Noyes, F.R., Zernicke, R.F., Biomechanics of ligaments and tendons. Exerc. Sport Sci. Rev. 6:125–182, 1978.

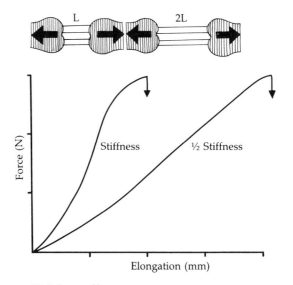

Figure 1-9. *Effect of length on tendon behavior. The longer tendon is stretched less at the same load application; thus less physical deformation takes place. Redrawn with permission from Butler, D.L., Grood, E.S., Noyes, F.R., Zernicke, R.F. Biomechanics of ligaments and tendons.* Exerc. Sport Sci. Rev. *6:125–182, 1978.*

amount of elongation, known as *strain*, that has occurred. The result is the familiar *stress-strain curve* (Fig. 1-10), which is similar in appearance to the load-elongation curve but is independent of physical dimensions.

Time

All connective tissues, including tendon, are viscoelastic; that is, they exhibit both fluid and solid properties. Thus the mechanical behavior of tendon is rate-dependent as well as size-dependent. For example, the rate at which force is applied plays a large role in the amount of force that the tendon can withstand. The rate of the tendon's lengthening is usually referred to as the strain rate, or the rate of deformation. Characteristically, tendons and ligaments can withstand larger forces when the forces are applied rapidly.

Another time-dependent feature of connective tissue is relaxation. If a tissue is stretched rapidly until a certain level of strain is reached and then is maintained at this fixed length while the force is measured, this force is seen to decrease over time (Fig. 1-11) until an equilibrium point is reached. Conversely, if a load is applied rapidly and maintained while the length is allowed to vary, the tissue lengthens with time (Fig. 1-12).

When a soft-tissue specimen is deformed at a constant rate and then allowed to return to its original length at the same rate while the force is monitored, there is a difference in the two curves; that is, less force is borne at the same length. This represents a loss of energy during the loading process, usually in the form of heat. This phenomenon is called *hysteresis* (Fig. 1-13).

The properties of relaxation, creep, and hysteresis are all features of viscoelastic materials. Although it is not essential to know them by name, the principles illustrated are very important in understanding concepts presented later in this book. A simple example will illustrate the points just mentioned. If, in stretching the hamstring

---

1. Normal tendon

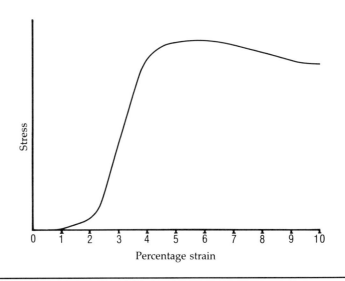

Figure 1-10. Stress-strain curve for the tendon.

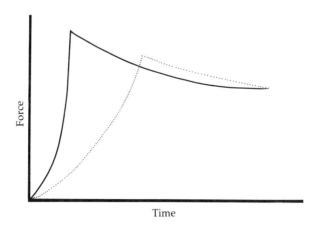

Figure 1-11. A force-time curve demonstrating that the tension "relaxes" (bears less load) after elongation to a fixed length.

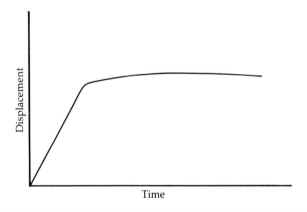

Figure 1-12. A length-time curve showing that the tendon lengthens with time at a constant load, a phenomenon called creep.

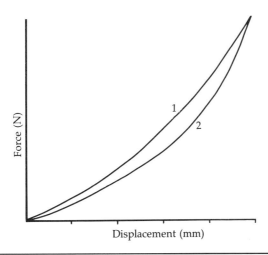

Figure 1-13. The difference between the slopes of the two curves shown here represents a loss of energy during the loading process. This is known as hysteresis.

muscle group, we apply a stretch (tensile force) and maintain it, then the soft tissue will elongate with time because of the property of relaxation. Also some heat will be released. This may partially explain why gentle stretching exercises can be used to warm up muscles.

Metabolic activity
For many years tendon was mistakenly assumed to be metabolically inert except in growing animals. It is true that tendon is much less active than such tissues as muscle or liver. Gerber et al. (1960a) measured the rates of turnover of rat collagen in various tissues and found that of tendon collagen to be 50 to 100 days, as compared with 50 days for muscle and 30 days for liver. If we compare these rates to that of actively growing tissue (for example, 1 to 2 days in the uterus during pregnancy), then the rate does seem slow.

Growth of collagen involves a balance between two processes: synthesis and degradation. During growth or following injury, synthesis exceeds breakdown, and the total amount of collagen increases. When growth ceases, the two are balanced.

Landi et al. (1980a,b,c) found in rabbits that enzymes of both the anaerobic and oxidative pathways decreased with age, with oxidative activity ceasing at maturity. They interpreted this as indicating a decreased potential for biosynthesis, or repair. Interestingly, levels of these enzymes increased following injury and decreased as healing took place.

A number of factors can affect the metabolism of collagen: altered gene expression, hormones, nutrition, nervous control, drugs, exercise, and so on. Genetic factors may govern the number of cells in a given tissue and the amount of protein produced by these cells. Many connective-tissue disorders are genetically determined. Hormones such as corticosteroids inhibit the production of new collagen and promote the removal of already formed collagen. Insulin, testosterone, and estrogen, however, have the opposite effect. Vitamin

---

1. Normal tendon

C is vital for collagen synthesis. Deficiencies in this vitamin cause failure in protein production by fibroblasts and may even induce their reversal to more immature cell types. Similarly, decreased levels of vitamin A and of many B vitamins result in decreased collagen synthesis.

Since proteins are composed of amino acids, an adequate supply of these via dietary protein is necessary. Carbohydrates are also important in forming the ground substance.

The role of nervous activity in the control of protein synthesis remains unclear. Muscle and tendon atrophy and their collagen content decreases when their nerve supply is interrupted. However, these changes also occur during immobilization and may be at least partly due to mechanical causes. Inactivity results in increased collagen degradation (Vailas et al. 1981), decreased tensile strength (Tipton et al. 1975), and decreased concentration of metabolic enzymes (Vailas et al. 1978). Exercise, however, increases collagen synthesis and concentration of metabolic enzymes, the fibers' size and number, and their tensile strength (Booth and Gould 1975).

Clearly, tendon and other connective tissues are metabolically active despite earlier misconceptions. Only recently has research interest in this area been renewed, because of the long-held belief that metabolic activity was so low as to be almost unappreciable, and healing slow and imperfect. Therefore, the roles of the various factors mentioned here remain to be determined.

Blood supply

Tendon is described in many textbooks as an avascular tissue in explanation of its slow rate of healing. However, it is avascular only relative to such tissue as muscle and skin.

Most authors seem to agree that a tendon receives its blood supply via three routes (although this agreement does not extend to the rel-

---

1. Normal tendon

ative importance of each): the musculotendinous junction, along the length of the tendon, and the bone-tendon junction. The musculotendinous and tendon-bone vessels are responsible for the distal thirds of the tendon, respectively, while the vessels from the paratenon or synovial sheath supply the central third.

The musculotendinous junction

A number of longitudinal vessels traverse the musculotendinous junction, but these are found only in the superficial covering of the muscle (perimysium). The capillary circulation of muscle and tendon is completely separate, in keeping with the lack of continuity between the muscle and tendon fibers. The capillaries adjacent to the musculotendinous junction loop back into the muscle or tendon, and there are no anastomoses between them. There are, however, small vessels that divide near the musculotendinous junction and supply branches to both muscle and tendon.

The length of the tendon

The blood supply here is from either the paratenon (the thin, filmy layer of areolar tissue covering the tendon) or the synovial sheath (which replaces the paratenon where the tendon is subjected to friction). The paratenon contains many vessels which are largely responsible for the tendon's blood supply, particularly (perhaps even solely) the middle third. Small branches from vessels in the paratenon run transversely toward the tendon and branch several times before assuming a course parallel to the tendon's long axis. Where tendons are invested with a synovial sheath, the paratenon continues, between two layers of synovial tissue, as the mesotenon. The circulation in the visceral layer of the tenosynovium communicates with the tendon.

Many authors ascribe great importance to the blood supply along the length of the tendon and relate the incidence of tendinitis to zones of decreased vasculature. This is one of the proposed etiologic

1. Normal tendon

factors in supraspinatus tendinitis of the shoulder (MacNab 1973), and it has been implicated in Achilles tendinitis as well (Smart, Taunton, and Clement 1980; Clancy 1982). Since healing is affected by blood flow and much of the tendon appears to be solely dependent on this source of blood supply, this may be an important etiologic factor.

The tendon-bone junction

The vessels of tendon and bone do not communicate directly because the tendon fibers gradually convert to fibrocartilage near the osseotendinous junction. There are, however, indirect anastomoses between tendon vessels and those of the periosteum. This source of blood supply supplies up to one-third of the tendon.

Internal vasculature

The blood vessels within the tendon are oriented primarily longitudinally in the endotenon and thus are arranged around the fascicles. These vessels, arteriolar in size, are flanked by two veins. Capillaries loop from the arterioles to the venules but do not penetrate the collagen bundles. The internal system, aligned in the tendon's long axis, is fed by vessels in the epitenon which branch and enter the tendon radially via the endotenon.

The vasculature of the tendon is variable and is reduced in areas of friction, torsion, compression, or excessive wear. We develop this concept further in Chapter 2 when we discuss its relationship to tendinitis.

Innervation of tendon

The nerve supply to the tendon is sensory and is derived from the appropriate overlying nerve. Normally, proprioceptive information that is picked up via sensory nerve endings near the musculotendinous junction is relayed to the central nervous system. There are

1. Normal tendon

23

two broad categories of mechanoreceptors: the Golgi tendon organ (GTO) and lamellated corpuscles (Bistevins and Awad 1981). Both are found within 1 cm of the musculotendinous junction. The GTO responds primarily to tension within the tendon such as that produced during muscle contraction or passive stretch. The lamellated corpuscles respond to stimuli transmitted via the surrounding tissue, such as pressure, which also may be produced by muscle contraction. Since the amount of pressure depends on the force of the contraction, the lamellated corpuscles may provide more finely tuned feedback.

Summary

In this chapter we have reviewed the anatomy, physiology, and mechanics of tendon. This is intended as groundwork for the ensuing discussion of tendinitis and of the role of exercise in its treatment, but it is by no means a complete discussion. Readers wishing further detail are urged to consult any of several excellent reviews listed in the References, most notably those of Viidik (1973) and Butler et al. (1978). However, the material in this chapter, although abbreviated, will provide you with an understanding of tendon's basic structure and function.

1. Normal tendon

2. *Tendinitis*

Tendon, like other soft tissues, is susceptible to injury from a variety of sources: direct blows, excessive tensile force, even breaks or tears. The body's response to any injury is the "inflammatory response," followed by repair. *Tendinitis* is the word used to describe inflammation of a tendon.

Most tendon injuries fall into the classification known as *overuse syndromes*. Also, because tendons have a less rich blood supply than other soft tissues such as skin or muscle (see Chapter 1), they are slower in healing. In this chapter, we discuss the common causes of tendinitis, describe the changes that occur during injury and healing, and review some of the methods of treatment.

Etiology: the mechanics of tendon injury

The term *overuse* means that the tendon has been loaded repeatedly until it is unable to withstand further loading, at which point damage occurs. Even the strongest of materials, such as steel, fatigues after repeated loads, even if individually these loads are well within the material's strength limits.

Tendon is remarkably strong: its tensile strength is 49 to 98 N/mm^2 (Elliott 1965). Most values for force and stress in the literature are given in kilograms or kilograms per square millimeter; however, the correct units are newtons (N) or pascals (Pa). Thus, the value we cite from Elliott (1965) is more properly stated in units of stress, or 49 to 98 MPa. Throughout this book, we use the correct units, which means that most values cited have been converted to these units from their original ones. There is a large gap between the stress that causes tendon failure and physiologic loads. The latter are reported to produce less than 4 percent strain (Elliott 1965). This is the "safe" zone of the stress-strain curve (see Fig. 1-7, p. 11), and it represents the straightening of the crimped collagen fibers when tendon is perfectly elastic and recovers its original length after the load is removed. Using muscles from rabbit hind legs, Elliott (1965) found that tendons of fusiform muscles transmit a maximum tension of no greater than 25 MPa, whereas those of pennate muscles transmit less than 15 MPa (Fig. 2-1). Both he and Walker et al. (1964) suggested that tendon is probably never stressed to greater than one-quarter of its ultimate tensile strength during normal activities.

The muscle force may be replaced by two perpendicular vectors (represented by arrows in Fig. 2-1), with one oriented in the tendon's long axis. The size of each vector is determined by the angle of orientation of the muscle fibers. The lateral components largely cancel each other if both parts of pennate muscle are equally active, leaving a tensile force to be applied to the tendon in series with the muscle. Pennate muscles, therefore, exert less tensile force on the tendon because of the greater angle between the longitudinal axes of the muscle and the tendon. This is true even though the muscle fibers of fusiform and pennate muscles are capable of producing equal amounts of force (Alexander and Vernon 1975b).

There are few studies in which the tensile forces have been estimated at the time of injury. Zernicke, Garhammer, and Jobe (1977) estimated a force of approximately 17 times the body weight acting on the patellar tendon of a skilled weight lifter at the moment of tendon rupture. For a 71-kg man whose tendon is assumed to have a cross-sectional area of 200 mm^2, or 2 cm^2, the stress on the tendon would be 29.6 MPa. This load is certainly larger than one-quarter the values cited by Elliott (1965). Indeed, during kicking, forces of up to 5200 N (26 MPa) have been estimated (Wahrenberg, Lindbeck, and Ekholm 1978), leading these authors to suggest that such forces, if repeated, may damage the patellar tendon. Given adequate time following such stresses, the tendon can recover, but reapplying force before this recovery has taken place may lead to injury.

---

2. Tendinitis

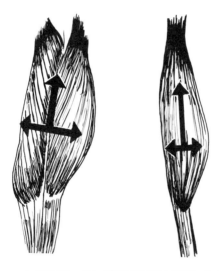

Figure 2-1. The force produced by a muscle can be resolved into two vectors, one in the long axis of the muscle or limb and the other perpendicular to it. The lateral vector is really the sum of two vectors, as shown here. Pennate muscles have obliquely oriented fibers, which means that more of their force is laterally directed than that of fusiform muscles (right). Since these vectors cancel, the vertical force on the tendon is seen to be less for pennate muscles, as noted by Elliott (1965) and Alexander (1974).

Most tests of tendon tensile strength are performed under nonphysiologic conditions, by using isolated tendon specimens and subjecting them to purely tensile loading. Tendons are rarely stressed this simply in vivo. According to Barfred (1971), in a survey of the anatomy, physiology, and mechanics of the bone-muscle-tendon group in general, tendon is most vulnerable when (1) tension is applied quickly, (2) tension is applied obliquely, (3) the tendon is tense before the trauma, (4) the attached muscle is maximally innervated, (5) the muscle group is stretched by exterior stimuli, or (6) the tendon is weak in comparison with the muscle. These situations occur commonly in athletics where maximum effort is made, movement is incertain or unexpected, or gravity or an opposing muscle stretches a contracting muscle. The variety of circumstances that can occur during sports means that while much valuable information can be gained from experimental studies, the extrapolation of results to the athletic environment remains largely hypothetical.

Elliott (1965) mentions that in cases of injury one should look for an alteration in the normally straight angle between the bone of insertion and the muscle belly. This may lead to an unequal distribution of stress in parts of the tendon that would then form the most likely sites of rupture. An example is the twisting of the Achilles tendon during its course through the leg to insert on the calcaneus (see Chapter 4).

Pathology—what happens to the tendon?

Tendon in the resting state has a wavy configuration, which appears as regular bands across the surface of the tendon (Fig. 2-2). When the tendon is stretched, the wave pattern disappears. The disappearance of the wave pattern means that the collagen fibers have been straightened. Provided that the tendon has not been stretched more than 4 percent, it will immediately resume its normal appearance if the force is released.

---

2. Tendinitis

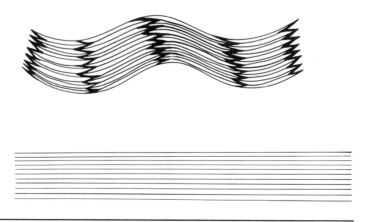

Figure 2-2. Straightening of the crimped fibrils.

If larger loads are applied and the tendon is elongated more than 4 percent, then the collagen fibers themselves are subjected to stress. This corresponds to region II of the stress-strain curve (Fig. 1-7). The size and number of the collagen fibrils will determine the amount of force that can be applied before damage occurs. At 4 to 8 percent strain, the collagen fibrils slide past one another; at 8 to 10 percent strain, the tendon begins to fail and resists less force. First, some of the cross links between neighboring molecules break (Fig. 2-3). Because of tendon's uniaxial composite structure, the force is shared and individual fibers are less likely to be overloaded (as long as they are linked to their neighbors). As more and more cross links are broken, the weakest fibers rupture and the tendon loses its composite structure. This increases the load on those remaining fibers. Continued application of force results in sequential fiber failure and, ultimately, rupture of the tendon.

Since even the largest physiologic loads fall within the limit of 12 percent strain, the changes that occur during tendinitis probably take place primarily at the molecular level and so are not visible to the eye. In addition, the sliding of the fibrils and the interposed matrix may cause a shearing force which can damage the tendon microvasculature. The reduction in vascular supply is important, since this is the vehicle by which oxygen and other nutrients reach the interior of the tendon. Oxygen is especially important because it is essential in establishing the cross links between the tropocollagen molecules.

The injured tendon, therefore, is one with microscopic or macroscopic damage to both its structural units and its blood supply. In this state, the tendon is predisposed to further injury since time is required for healing to take place. This healing begins with the inflammatory response and is usually accompanied by pain, the first clinical sign of tendinitis.

---

2. Tendinitis

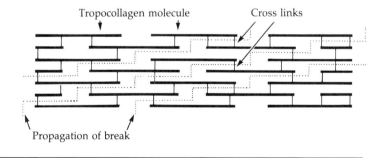

Figure 2-3. Tropocollagen molecules are held together by intramolecular and intermolecular bonds, or cross links. As these bonds break, the process spreads through the remaining tendon molecules.

Tendon healing

Tendon, like other soft tissues, heals in stages. An understanding of these stages is important, since the physical and chemical environment during each stage affects the healing process. Most studies of connective-tissue healing have been done on incisional wounds, where the tendon or skin has been completely divided. These are not the best models for healing in clinical tendinitis, where damage is usually microscopic. Nevertheless, the principles remain the same, with the difference lying only in the degree of the response.

Connective-tissue healing is divided into two broad stages: *proliferative* and *formative* (Chvapil 1967). During the former, which lasts approximately 14 days, cells migrate to the area and new connective tissue is laid down. This new tissue is remodeled during the formative stage, which extends from the end of the proliferative stage until the tissue is as near normal as possible.

Chvapil (1967) further subdivides connective-tissue healing (which he calls *fibroproductive inflammation*) into four stages:

1. Cell mobilization (inflammatory response)
2. Ground substance proliferation
3. Collagen protein formation
4. Final organization

Stages 1 to 3 are the proliferative stage of healing. We use this classification since it correlates readily with the treatment program outlined later.

Cell mobilization (inflammatory response)

The damage to the tendon microvasculature that occurs at the time of injury results in bleeding and increased permeability of the remaining intact vessels, so that fluid accumulates in the area (if the area is large, this is readily seen as swelling around the tendon). The rupture of damaged cells releases chemicals that initiate this increase in vessel permeability (vasodilatation) and that act as signals to other

2. Tendinitis

cells to come to the area to aid in cleaning up the damaged tissue. Some of the chemicals released help break down the connective-tissue elements.

The inflammatory response begins when injury occurs and lasts about 48 hours. Although it may seem destructive rather than reparative, it is necessary to draw cells involved with the healing process to the area, such as white blood cells. Eliminating the inflammatory response by drug administration can delay or interrupt healing.

Although the inflammatory response is necessary to initiate healing, it should last only a short time. Hypoxia results from impaired circulation caused by stasis of the extracellular fluid, and the acidic environment in the area of injury causes an increase in proteolytic activity, which may be detrimental to the surrounding healthy connective tissue if the inflammation is prolonged.

Ground substance proliferation

The ground substance is the gellike matrix that surrounds the collagen fibrils, and it is composed of proteins, carbohydrates, and water. Ground substance is produced by the fibroblasts, which are found in the surrounding connective tissue. The existence of an adequate amount of ground substance is necessary for the aggregation of collagenous proteins (which also are produced by the fibroblasts) into the shape of fibrils. This stage takes place until day 3 or 4.

Collagen protein formation

Until day 5 following the injury, a high proportion of collagen is soluble, or immature, because cross links have not yet formed between the tropocollagen molecules. Soluble collagen is much more susceptible to breakdown by enzymes that the inflammatory response activates (hence the importance of limiting the inflammation after the initial phase of the injury). From day 6 to day 14, the proportion of

2. Tendinitis

insoluble collagen increases as cross links form between the tropocollagen molecules. The rate of collagen degradation concomitantly decreases, since cross-linked collagen resists enzymatic degradation.

Final organization

From day 14 onward, collagen continues to increase and begins to organize into fibrils that are laid down randomly. Tension now begins to play an important role in the healing process because the collagen fibers reorient themselves in line with the tensile force applied to the tissue. In fact, the rate of collagen fiber formation is directly related to the functional state of the affected area. The amount of tension that is necessary or optimal remains unclear. All tendons are subjected to some tension through contraction of their attached muscles, but the amount may be markedly reduced if joint motion is prevented.

Stress on the collagen fibers also produces a piezoelectric effect, resulting in the development of an electric potential. Since collagen molecules have an electric charge, this may affect their alignment as well and may be a means by which tension helps reorient the collagen fibrils. The use of electric stimulation to enhance tendon healing, in a manner similar to techniques now used to promote fracture healing, is just beginning to receive attention.

Forms of treatment

The variation in locations of tendinitis, together with the lack of agreement as to etiology in many cases (or even exact location), has led to a bewildering assortment of treatment techniques. Most are based on scientific principles but are not equally well adapted to different patients. For example, a retired man with tennis elbow may respond more readily to the suggestion of rest as a form of therapy than a young volleyball player with jumper's knee who is in the middle of the season. These factors must be considered when a form

2. Tendinitis

of treatment is chosen, since patient compliance is the single largest factor determining the success or failure of treatment.

We feel that treatment can be divided, broadly, into rest and activity. However, because many forms of treatment are combined with both rest and activity, we have modified this classification somewhat and present it in the form shown in Table 2-1.

Rest

Rest may mean anything from briefly stopping any pain-causing activity to having the affected limb placed in a cast for 3 to 6 weeks. In general, if an activity causes pain of such magnitude that one cannot perform the activity, then it is wise to stop that activity *for a short time.* This is only common sense and appears even more logical if we consider that pain is a clinical sign of the inflammatory reaction of tissue and thus acts as a warning signal.

Table 2-1. Forms of treatment for tendinitis

Treatment	Used in this stage of healing
Rest	1, 2, 3
Stop activity	
Cast immobilization	
Taping/support	1, 2, 3, 4
Physical modalities	1, 2, 3
Ice	
Electric stimulation	
"Deep heat"	
Ultrasound	
Drugs	1, 2, 3
Anti-inflammatories (oral)	
Steroids (injection)	
Exercise	3, 4
Stretching	
Strengthening	
Surgery	1 (rupture) or 4 (chronic)

2. Tendinitis

Equally, if a person ceases, permanently, to participate in an activity that produces pain or discomfort, then it is likely that he or she will no longer suffer that discomfort. This is unacceptable to most athletes and economically impossible for patients whose tendinitis is related to their occupation.

Cast immobilization for long periods is unnecessary and undesirable from both a physiologic and a mechanical point of view. During joint immobilization, tendons lose from 20 to 40 percent of their ground substance (Akeson, Amiel, and LaViolette 1967), and new connective tissue formed during periods of immobility may contain less elastin. Furthermore, the removal of mechanical influences on the newly formed collagen means that orientation of the collagen fibrils cannot take place, and they are laid down randomly, which reduces the tensile strength of the healing tendon. Those fibers not subjected to tension are resorbed in the remodeling process, which continues until the tissue's collagen content returns to normal. For this reason, inactivity is to be discouraged after day 14 following the injury, since it is detrimental to collagen fiber orientation and to tendon strength, which depends on the number, size, and orientation of the fibers. In addition to the effects on the injured tendon itself, immobilization has profound effects on muscles and other soft tissues in the immobilized limb. Muscle wasting and weakness, joint stiffness, and lack of proprioception occur in other areas besides those injured. Thus after cast removal a great deal of rehabilitation may be necessary to return an athlete to competition.

For these reasons, we do not advocate cast immobilization of injured tendons. If rest is necessary, withdrawal from the sport may be advised for 1 to 2 days (longer if necessary). Alternatively, limited rest may be achieved through the use of taping, elastic supports, or braces (Fig. 2-4). The concept of limited rest means that the injured tendon is used but is protected from stress which may damage it further. The use of measures such as those of Figure 2-4 should *always* be augmented by a program designed to correct the initial cause of the tendinitis.

2. Tendinitis

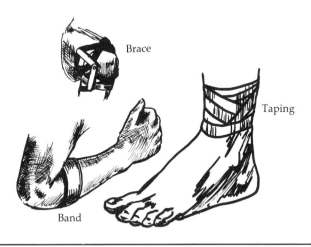

Brace

Taping

Band

Figure 2-4. Some devices may assist the athlete by restricting motion to a nonpainful range.

Drugs

NONSTEROIDAL   We have mentioned both the importance of the inflammatory reaction in initiating healing and the desirability of limiting this reaction if it is prolonged beyond its normal time limits (1 to 2 days). Note that this period is the same as that advised for rest in cases of acute tendinitis.

The prescription of any drug is, of course, done by the physician. There are a variety of types and brand names, which need not be mentioned here. The individual physician prescribes what he or she feels to be most suitable.

Aspirin is a potent anti-inflammatory drug and is available without prescription. Its use is convenient in cases where pain is not intense or where symptoms fluctuate. Nonetheless, the patient should obtain advice on dosage from a professional before self-administering any drug.

CORTICOSTEROIDS   Steroids are also anti-inflammatory drugs, and injections of these drugs are not uncommonly used in the treatment of tendinitis. There are numerous reports in the literature, however, of tendon ruptures following steroid injection (Halpern, Horowitz, and Nagel 1977; Unverferth and Olix 1973; Sweetnam 1969). Experimental studies have shown that the tensile strength of the tendon is decreased following steroid injection and that the production of collagen and ground substance is reduced (Wrenn et al. 1954; Kennedy and Baxter-Willis 1976). Degenerative changes occur in both the tendon and the paratenon, and the physical presence of the drug causes circulatory stasis, which is detrimental to the tendon's microvasculature.

Corticosteroid injection is especially contraindicated in the middle third of the tendon (where the blood supply may be wholly dependent on vessels from the paratenon) and in cases where continued physical activity is expected (or suspected), since this will increase

2. Tendinitis

the risk of rupture. The latter instance would involve any athletic activities and even normal walking for cases of Achilles tendinitis and jumper's knee.

If corticosteroid injection is employed, it should be placed into the tendon sheath only and followed by ice application to decrease the inflammatory reaction at the injection site. Physical activity should be reduced for 2 to 3 weeks. Since such injections frequently improve symptoms dramatically on a temporary basis, it is unlikely that the patient will refrain from activity, and the athlete may return to training, competition, or work prematurely.

Although some authors have failed to find any deleterious effects associated with steroid injection, the overwhelming majority are of the opposite opinion and discourage the use of steroids in treating tendinitis. In light of the known biochemical and mechanical effects, all of which are negative, we support this view.

Physical modalities

Physiotherapists treat tendinitis with such physical measures as ultrasound, short-wave diathermy or other forms of "deep heat," electric stimulation, massage, heat, cold, and whirlpool.

Cold decreases inflammation by reducing the rate of chemical activity and the vasoconstriction caused by brief periods of ice application (5 to 15 minutes). This should decrease swelling in the area as a result of increased permeability of the dilated capillaries. Cold is also an effective analgesic, decreasing sensory nerve conduction for 0.5 to 2 hours after application. The safest and most effective method of applying cold therapy is by means of crushed ice in a damp towel; however, immersion in ice water is also very effective. There are also numerous other means of applying cold therapy. Ice should be applied for a limited time (less than 15 minutes) and repeated every 1 to 2 hours in acute cases. For cases of chronic tendinitis, ice should be applied after any activity that produces discomfort.

---

2. Tendinitis

In ultrasound therapy, high-frequency sound waves are used to produce a mechanical effect on newly formed scar tissue. The piezoelectric effect is again at work, but this time in the opposite direction (i.e., an electric signal received by the sound head causes a crystal to vibrate, producing mechanical waves). The application of these waves renders the tissue more susceptible to subsequent remodeling by appropriate tensile forces. Thus ultrasound usually should be followed by exercise. Ultrasound can have a heating effect also and is believed by many physiotherapists to reduce inflammation. This latter claim, however, has no real scientific basis, since it has not been proved experimentally.

Deep heat is a term that refers to any means by which heat is concentrated at a tissue level below the skin surface. It has the same effect as local heat application (increased temperature and blood flow). It may also reduce the stiffness of the connective tissue, making it a useful preliminary to stretching exercises.

The use of electric stimulation—transcutaneous neurologic stimulation (TNS or TENS)—is becoming more and more commonplace. Put most simply, it replaces the pain signal with a new one—an electric current. Pain relief lasts for varying lengths of time, depending on the severity of the symptoms. Since this treatment (as currently used) affects only the symptoms of tendinitis, other measures must be taken to eliminate the cause of the problem. One potentially interesting application of electric stimulation has already been alluded to—that of improving healing. Electric stimulation of healing fractures has become an accepted form of therapy, and electric stimulation of muscles to increase strength is commonly used also. At the Nova Scotia Sport Medicine Clinic, we have applied electric stimulation to healing surgically repaired dog anterior cruciate ligaments and found the stimulated ligaments to have greater tensile strength than the controls.

Massage is another popular physiotherapeutic maneuver to treat tendinitis. It refers to a technique called *deep frictions*, which is used

---

2. Tendinitis

to break down scar tissue. It is very uncomfortable, but effective when properly done by a skilled therapist.

Surgery

In patients whose tendinitis has been resistant to other forms of treatment, surgery is sometimes resorted to. The usual reason is to remove the buildup of scar tissue that accompanies repeated trauma and to encourage revascularization. This scar tissue usually forms as a result of increased collagen synthesis in response to injury, but is immature and disorganized, so that it adds little to the strength of the tendon. The removal of scar is followed by suturing of the tendon or leaving it to heal in a lengthened state (as in many cases of tennis elbow). Some form of postsurgical immobilization is usually required.

Although surgical intervention is unquestionably necessary following spontaneous tendon rupture, its value in cases of chronic tendinitis is less certain. Because surgery is usually followed by immobilization, an extended period of rest, and rehabilitation exercises, it is difficult to ascertain to what the clinical improvement is actually due. Surgery may be indicated in rare instances in which nonsurgical measures fail to effect any improvement in the patient's symptoms. The role of surgery could be better evaluated if controlled clinical trials were performed in which different groups of patients with the same diagnosed disorder received different forms of therapy, surgery included. This would allow a direct comparison of methods; however, it is seldom done.

Exercise

The role of activity in tendon healing was touched on earlier in this chapter when we discussed the importance of tension in the orientation of newly forming collagen fibrils. Increases in the size and mass of bone and muscle with activity, and their wasting with inactivity, have been recognized for many years. Indeed, most rehabili-

2. Tendinitis

tation programs are devoted to reversing the weakness and atrophy that follow injury or immobilization.

More recently, investigators have observed the same effects of use and disuse on ligaments and tendons. Noyes et al. (1974) studied the mechanical properties of anterior cruciate ligaments of monkeys after 8 weeks of cast immobilization and found a 39 percent decrease in maximum failure load and decreased stiffness. Even after 20 weeks of postimmobilization reconditioning the ligament had only partially recovered. In the same study, localized exercise was shown to be of no benefit in preventing weakening of the ligament during cast immobilization, leading these authors to suggest that localized exercise cannot reproduce and simulate the total force placed on an extremity in a normal ambulatory state. Swine trained for 12 months showed increases in stiffness, ultimate load, and total weight of extensor tendons (Woo et al. 1975), and Barfred (1971) noted that wild rats had much stronger ligaments than domesticated rats. Numerous other studies on rats (Tipton et al. 1967; Zuckerman and Stull 1973) and dogs (Tipton et al. 1970) show the same results—activity strengthens ligaments and tendons, inactivity weakens them.

Woo et al. (1975) showed that chronic exercise increases both the mechanical properties (material composition) and the structural properties (hypertrophy) of the tendon. A number of mechanisms have been implicated in the changing of connective-tissue properties: (1) changes in the synthesis and degradation equilibrium of collagen; (2) changes in collagen cross links on an intermolecular and intramolecular level; (3) alterations in water and electrolyte content of connective tissues; (4) changes in arrangement, number, and thickness of collagen fibers (Noyes et al. 1974). Mechanical stresses on the connective tissue must be necessary, since rats in a swimming training program do not show the same increases in ligament strength as those placed on a treadmill running program (A.C. Vailas, personal communication).

---

2. *Tendinitis*

One drawback of the experimental results just described is that they were all from studies involving animals. It is difficult, if not impossible, at present to perform similar experiments on human subjects, since they are reluctant to volunteer to have large ligament or tendon specimens removed! The development of miniaturized strain gauge techniques may make feasible the in vivo testing of human tendon, an area in which much research is needed but which remains virtually unexplored.

Summary

The application of force to the tendon via muscle contraction produces tensile stress in the attached tendon. The amount of stress is related to the magnitude of the force generated by the muscle, the direction of the force application, and the physical dimensions of the tendon. The most likely etiology for tendinitis is disruption of the tendon's structural integrity by tensile stresses that exceed the strength limits of some of the smaller fibrils or fibers. On a large scale, this may result in actual tendon rupture.

Tendon healing proceeds through two stages. During the first (proliferative) stage, new collagen is produced. A variety of physical modalities and rest are used to control the clinical symptoms (primarily pain) during this period. Next is the formative stage, in which tissue remodeling occurs. During this stage, which lasts until the collagen content and tendon structure are near normal, tensile stress should be introduced to optimize healing, since tension appears to play an important part in directing the organization of the new tissue.

The role of exercise in the form of tensile stress for treatment of soft-tissue disorders is firmly supported experimentally by animal studies. The results of such studies form the theoretical basis for the exercise program that forms the cornerstone of our therapeutic program. The rest of this book is devoted to the description of this program and its application to various tendon disorders.

2. *Tendinitis*

3. Exercise and the muscle-tendon unit

In the first chapters we presented the groundwork for understanding tendon structure, behavior under normal and abnormal circumstances, and methods of healing. In this chapter we consider the relationship between exercise and the tendon.

We know that muscles become stronger if they are exercised; if muscles are stretched, they become longer. But more than muscle, however, responds to exercise. Because of the functional integrity of muscle-tendon units, exercise also affects the tendons. Yet for many years this fact was ignored, owing to the continuing belief that tendons were mere inert bands of connective tissue.

The recent interest in tendons (and ligaments) has stimulated investigations into the effects of exercise on these structures. Here we explore this subject in detail.

Type of exercise

The basis for movement and exercise is muscle contraction. Characteristically we tend to regard contraction as a shortening of the muscle which occurs as the thick (myosin) and thin (actin) filaments slide past one another. Yet during many activities the overall muscle length does not change, and in some cases it may actually lengthen. These differences in muscle behavior during activity have led to the classification of muscle contraction (or exercise) as concentric, eccentric, or isometric (see Fig. 3-1).

Isometric

When the shoulder muscles contract to counter the downward forces produced by carrying an object, the muscles are acting iso-

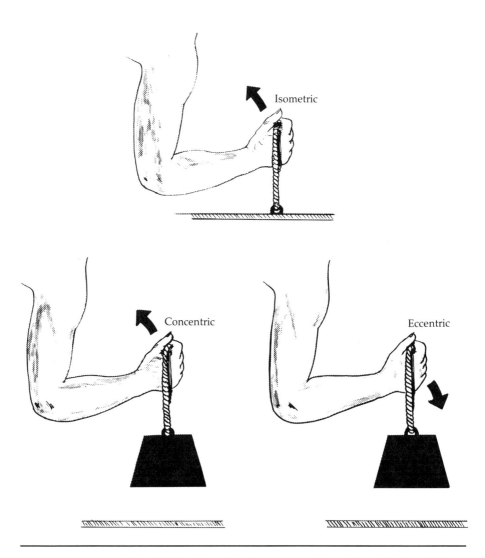

Figure 3-1. Three types of exercise: no movement occurs (isometric), the weight is lifted (concentric), the weight is lowered (eccentric).

metrically. Of course, no contraction is truly isometric, since some shortening *must* occur at the muscle fiber level. However, no change in the overall length of the muscle takes place. As a result, this type of contraction is referred to as *static*.

Concentric

During concentric contraction, muscles shorten while producing tension. Lifting weights against gravity makes use of this type of movement. In effect, the internal force generated by the muscles overcomes the force of the external resistance.

Eccentric

This kind of contraction is the opposite of a concentric one. When muscles contract eccentrically, they lengthen while producing force. The external resistance in this case is greater than the internal force produced by the muscles. Eccentric contractions are very common, since every movement in the direction of gravity is controlled by them, including sitting, descending stairs, and lowering weights. Also, most movements are preceded by a preliminary countermovement in the opposite direction; when direction is changed, eccentric contraction is usually involved.

Work and energy   All muscle contractions require energy to perform work. In order to produce energy, fuel must be consumed. Muscles generate mechanical energy, or work, by using the chemical energy ("fuel") produced from food. The processes of fuel transformation can proceed either with oxygen (aerobically) or without oxygen (anaerobically). Although these methods are very different, they both produce ATP (adenosine triphosphate), the chemical substance that allows muscles to contract. Eventually chemical energy becomes mechanical energy.

---

3. Exercise and the muscle-tendon unit

Mechanical work is the effect of applying a force to an object (be it a weight, a limb, or the body itself) and causing it to move. In the terms of the physicist or engineer, mechanical work is the product of force and distance. Muscles can perform two types of mechanical work: *positive* and *negative*.

Muscles accomplish positive work when they shorten and overcome an external resistance such as gravity. The potential energy of the system on which the muscles act increases, and the object being acted on moves in the same direction as the muscle contraction. Lifting a weight is a simple example of this type of work.

Negative work involves displacement of an object in an opposite (negative) direction to the force exerted by the muscles. In other words, movement is in the same direction as the external force. The muscles lengthen, and the potential energy of the system decreases. Lowering the weight just lifted is an example of negative work.

Potential energy is the energy due to gravity, and so it is the product of an object's weight (mass times acceleration due to gravity) and its height relative to the ground or some other suitable reference point. This is recognizable as nearly identical to the earlier definition of mechanical work. In positive work, when a muscle contracts to lift a weight, it produces more force than the force due to gravity acting on the object. The object's distance from the ground increases; so does its potential energy. In negative work, the muscle force is less than the force due to gravity (weight), and the potential energy decreases. These concepts are illustrated in Figure 3-2.

Positive work accelerates the body or limb. Negative work decelerates a moving object. In most cases, the terms *positive* and *negative* may be considered synonymous with *concentric* and *eccentric* contraction, respectively.

---

3. Exercise and the muscle-tendon unit

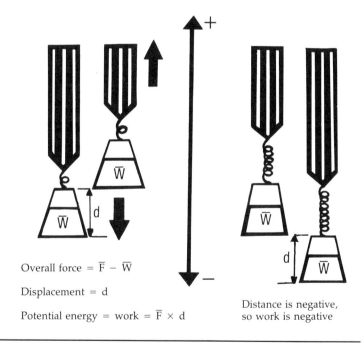

Overall force $= \overline{F} - \overline{W}$

Displacement $= d$

Potential energy $=$ work $= \overline{F} \times d$

Distance is negative,
so work is negative

Figure 3-2. Potential energy increases with positive work and decreases with negative work.

Force-velocity relationship

The force produced by skeletal muscle is dependent on both the speed of shortening and the length of the muscle at any instant in time. A typical curve of the relationship between velocity of muscle contraction and the force produced by the muscle is represented by Figure 3-3. This curve is similar for isolated muscle fibers, muscles involved in simple tasks such as elbow flexion (Wilkie 1950), or large muscle groups involved in more complex movements such as running or jumping.

The relationship between muscle force and speed of shortening differs for eccentric and concentric contraction. Figure 3-3 illustrates that in eccentric exercise, the force increases as the velocity of contraction increases (at least to a certain point). In contrast, during concentric exercise the force decreases as the speed of contraction increases.

The force-velocity relationship may have important applications to training. To increase muscle force under conditions of negative work (eccentric contraction), the limb should be moved as rapidly as possible. During concentric exercise, movement should be performed slowly to maximize force production. Figure 3-3 shows that the force production during eccentric contraction appears to be greater than during concentric exercise. Since this force is transmitted by the tendon to its insertion, the tendon is subjected to larger loads during eccentric exercise.

Although a great deal of literature is available on the force-velocity relationship during muscle shortening, unfortunately the same is not true of lengthening contractions, largely because of greater technical difficulty in experimental methods. Thus much of the current knowledge on muscle behavior during lengthening contractions is speculative, in many cases having been extrapolated from experimental results on concentric muscle action. This applies to the force-length relationship as well. More research is needed, especially on

3. Exercise and the muscle-tendon unit

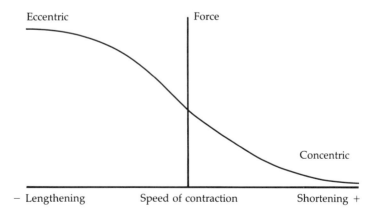

Figure 3-3. The force-velocity relationship for muscle (general case) showing that tension is higher during lengthening contractions and increases with speed of lengthening.

force-length and force-velocity relationships during actual activities, to determine the magnitudes of force production during eccentric as compared to concentric muscle work.

Force-time
relationship

To move efficiently, coordination between the signals for muscle contraction and force production is necessary. In sports, the mini-mization of time lags between these two is extremely important. There is a latent period of approximately 55 ms (Wood 1977) be-tween the signal for muscle contraction (from the brain) and the on-set of muscle electric (EMG) activity and a further delay between the appearance of EMG activity and tension in the muscle. Thus the sec-ond delay is referred to as the *electromechanical delay* (EMD) (Komi and Cavanaugh 1977). These authors have shown that EMD is shorter under conditions of eccentric contraction, suggesting that this is a strategy for producing the greatest force in the least time.

Force-length
relationship

When the joint between two adjusted bones changes its angle, so does the mechanical action of the muscle. This is a function of two variables: the length of the muscle and its distance from the joint center of rotation (see Fig. 3-4).

As muscles contract, they produce rotation at joints because the line of action of the muscle is located at a distance from the joint center of rotation. This distance is referred to as the *lever,* or *moment,* arm of the muscle. It is a line perpendicular to the muscle's line of action extending from that line to the joint center of rotation. The mathe-matical product of the force produced by the muscle and its moment arm is known as the *joint moment,* or *joint torque.* During most hu-man motion analysis, it is only this variable that can be estimated. The amount of force produced by muscles increases as the length of the muscle increases (up to a certain point). This increases the joint torque. The joint moment also increases if the distance between the

3. Exercise and the muscle-tendon unit

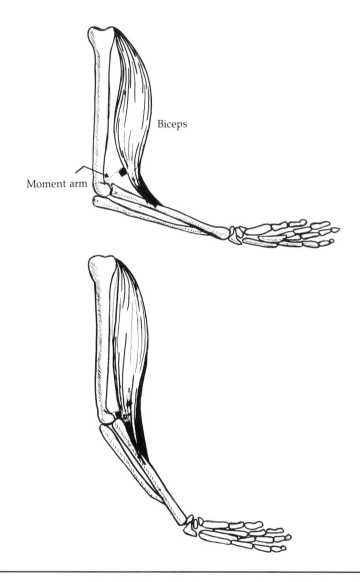

Biceps

Moment arm

Figure 3-4. The variation in moment arm (perpendicular distance between muscle and joint) and muscle length with elbow movement. Note that muscle length increases during extension, but the moment arm becomes much smaller. At 90°, however, the moment arm reaches a peak length. It is at this angle that the largest torque is produced.

muscle and the joint center of rotation increases. Thus, joint movement alters both the length and the moment arm of the muscle and thereby controls the joint moment. There is an optimum joint angle at which the product of force and moment arm is largest. As the joint moves away from this position, less torque is produced either because the muscle is too short (or too long) and thus produces less force or because the moment arm has become shorter. Most maximum joint torques occur at midrange. For example, the maximum joint torque at the elbow occurs at approximately 90° flexion. The relationship between joint angle and muscle force is shown in Figure 3-5.

For isolated muscle fibers, force production increases with length until a critical length is reached, then decreases because less filament overlap is possible. This relationship also holds for whole muscles but is complicated by alterations in the moment arm. Thus, the relationship between joint angle and force production is not simply the relationship between force and length, but involves change in the mechanical action that the muscle is able to exert on the joint.

Neurologic influences

Muscle contraction and force production are governed not only by mechanical factors such as length and lever arm, but also by the activity of the muscle. The basic component of the neuromuscular system is the motor unit—an anterior horn cell, its motor axon, and all the muscle fibers it innervates. There are varying numbers of motor units within the muscles. Muscle contraction can be graded by increasing either the number of motor units that are active at any particular time or the frequency of their firing. Differences in firing frequency have led to the designation of two motor unit types: slow twitch (ST) and fast twitch (FT). The latter are able to produce more force because they have higher firing frequencies and larger muscle fibers or more fibers per motor unit.

3. Exercise and the muscle-tendon unit

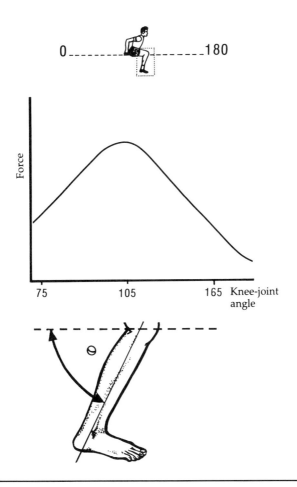

Figure 3-5. Variation in force as knee extends, because the moment arm decreases and the muscle shortens after midrange.

Muscle contraction is under both voluntary and reflex control. The muscle length and the force and speed of the contraction are monitored by sensory receptors in the muscle and tendon—the *muscle spindles* and the *Golgi tendon organs* (GTOs). The former provide feedback to the central nervous system concerning muscle length and velocity, while the GTO, located in the tendon near the musculotendinous junction, provides information about the force acting on the tendon. The signals from these two receptor types have opposite reflex effects on muscles (see Fig. 3-6). The muscle spindle signal tends to produce muscle shortening (since the spindles are stretched by elongation of the muscle, being parallel with it). The GTO is affected most by active muscle contraction and produces reflex relaxation of the muscle. The actions of the different receptors allow the muscle to respond to both passive and active lengthening or shortening and alter the "sensitivity" of the muscle, perhaps allowing it to produce more force at certain positions.

The preceding paragraphs describe neurologic control of the muscle-tendon unit in its simplest form and are included to illustrate the complex interaction that allows muscle force production to be modified. The reader is referred to other sources such as texts of neurophysiology for a more complete description.

Muscle elasticity | Basically, the muscle-tendon unit, despite its complexity, can be modeled as a two-component system: a contractile component (CC) in series with an elastic component (SEC) (Komi 1979). This model is represented in Figure 3-7A.

It is the rearrangement in length of the contractile and elastic muscle-tendon components that produces force in all three types of muscle contractions. In isometric contraction, force is generated by the contractile component and is accompanied by stretching of the series elastic component. In concentric contraction, some stretching of the SEC occurs, but most of the force is produced by the actual

3. *Exercise and the muscle-tendon unit*

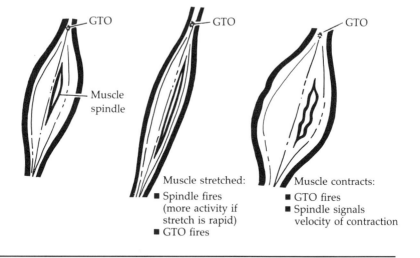

GTO

GTO

GTO

Muscle
spindle

Muscle stretched:
- Spindle fires
  (more activity if
  stretch is rapid)
- GTO fires

Muscle contracts:
- GTO fires
- Spindle signals
  velocity of contraction

Figure 3-6. Two types of muscle-tendon receptors and how they are affected.

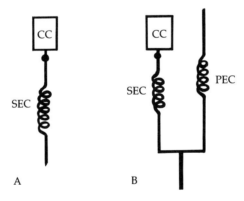

Figure 3-7. Theoretical models for muscle behavior. A. This is the simplest, with just a contractile component (CC) and series elastic component (SEC). B. This is slightly more complicated because a parallel elastic component (PEC) is shown in parallel with both the CC and SEC. This represents connective tissue such as muscle sheaths.

sliding of the muscle fiber filaments past one another. During eccentric contraction, the muscle is lengthening as it contracts, which stretches the SEC and allows it to contribute to force production.

The presence of the series elastic component may account for the high tension that occurs in eccentric contraction (see Fig. 3-8). The total force generated is the sum of that produced by contraction of the CC and by stretching of the SEC.

The actual location of the SEC is a matter of some controversy. Although most authors agree that the tendon, because it is in series with the muscle, must form at least part of the SEC, many believe that the major portion of the SEC resides in the myosin cross-bridges, which are stretched during that part of muscle contraction when the actin and myosin are in contact and moving away from each other. Other connective-tissue elements in parallel with the muscle also may contribute to force production at lengths far above the resting length. This is the parallel elastic component (PEC), illustrated in Figure 3-7B. The PEC is thought to play only a minor role in most physiologic activities (Thys, Faraggiana, and Margaria 1972).

In most movements, muscle action seldom begins from a static starting position. The push-off phase in running is preceded by the heel-strike and foot-flat phases. Similarly, a downward motion of the body, with knee flexion, almost always precedes the upward jumping motion in volleyball and basketball (in other words, an eccentric contraction of the quadriceps) (see Fig. 3-9).

Thus, in most sports activities, muscle is stretched before it contracts concentrically. This mechanism enhances muscle force production by stretching the SEC and allowing it to contribute. Reflex activity (via muscle spindles and GTOs) also may contribute to force production by increasing the stiffness of the muscle, that is, by making it "springier." Many researchers have shown that eccentric contraction enhances muscle force production and is less costly metaboli-

---

3. Exercise and the muscle-tendon unit

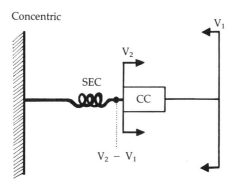

Concentric

V_1

V_2

SEC

CC

$V_2 - V_1$

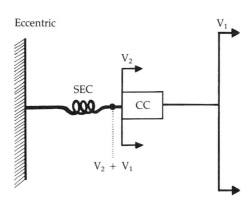

Eccentric

V_1

V_2

SEC

CC

$V_2 + V_1$

Figure 3-8. In concentric contraction, the velocity and force are contributed to by the CC only, since the muscle ends are moving to "unload" the SEC. The opposite is true in eccentric contractions—the SEC is stretched and contributes to force production. Redrawn with permission from Komi, P.V., Neuromuscular performance: factors influencing force and speed production. Scand. J. Sports Sci. 1:2–15, 1979.

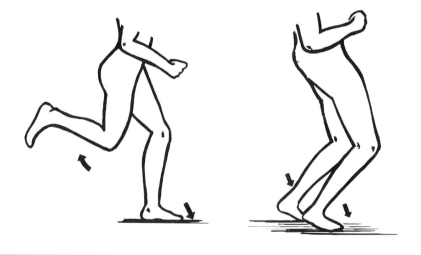

Figure 3-9. Eccentric contractions are required in both running and jumping.

cally than concentric contraction (Bosco and Komi 1979; Cavagna, Saibene, and Margaria 1965; Cavagna, Dusman, and Margaria 1968; Komi 1973, 1979; Komi and Bosco 1978; Thys, Faraggiana, and Margaria 1972). More force is produced at less metabolic expense as the body improves the efficiency of muscle contraction by using the "stored elastic energy" of the SEC.

Eccentric exercise program	The foregoing information was presented as scientific background for the program we use to treat tendinitis, which we call the *eccentric exercise program*. After careful questioning of many afflicted athletes, we began to realize that eccentric contraction was somehow involved in the production of tendinitis. In the case of a basketball player, for example, we discovered that the *exact* moment of greatest pain occurred in landing from a jump, although pain often would be felt during takeoff as well. Further testing revealed that in many cases pain could be reproduced in the clinic only by eccentric loading. If we refer to what we know about muscle-tendon mechanics, this seems logical. Greater force production during eccentric contraction translates into greater stress on the tendon during this type of activity.

Noting this relationship, we designed a training program that would (theoretically) strengthen the actual tendon tissue. We reasoned that the forces to which the tendon was subjected during activity were causing damage to the tendon microstructure at the collagen fiber level. Although various types of weight training programs were frequently part of the athlete's existing training program, the emphasis was usually on concentric or isokinetic exercises. We added eccentric exercises designed to reinforce the muscle-tendon unit and focused the training regimen on three functional areas:

1. *Length.* Stretching would be an integral part of the program. By increasing the resting length of the muscle-tendon unit, we could

---

3. Exercise and the muscle-tendon unit

lessen the strain (deformation) taking place during the same range of joint movement. Research has indicated that stretching may strengthen the tendon.

2. *Load.* Increasing the load would clearly subject the tendon to greater stress and would form the basis for the progression of the program. This principle of progressive overloading forms the basis of all physical training programs.

3. *Speed of contraction.* The force on the tendon is related to the speed of muscle contraction (see Fig. 3-9). Increasing the speed of the movement would also increase the load on the tendon.

Based on these factors, we developed the eccentric exercise program outlined here:

1. Stretch
   a. Static stretch
   b. Hold 15 to 30 seconds
   c. Repeat 3 to 5 times
2. Eccentric exercise
   a. Three sets of 10 repetitions
   b. Progression:
      Days 1 and 2: slow
      Days 3 to 5: moderate
      Days 6 and 7: fast
   c. Increase external resistance; after day 7, repeat cycle
3. Stretch, as prior to exercise.
4. Ice: crushed ice or ice massage applied to tender or painful area for 5 to 10 minutes

Pain

The presenting symptom of tendinitis is pain; indeed, that is why the athlete seeks help. Pain, which indicates ongoing inflammation in the tendon, is the most common measure used to classify the degree of tendinitis severity. We devised the following system of symptom classification, similar to that used by other authors (Fox et al. 1975; Perugia, Ippolito, and Postacchini 1976):

---

3. Exercise and the muscle-tendon unit

Level 1. No pain
Level 2. Pain only after extreme exertion
Level 3. Pain with extreme exertion and for 1 to 2 hours afterward
Level 4. Pain during and after vigorous activities
Level 5. Pain during activity that forces termination
Level 6. Pain during daily activities

Table 3-1 shows the effect of pain on athletic performance. Although pain is a subjective assessment, this classification of tendinitis severity can be a criterion for evaluation. We use the degree of reported pain, included in both the pre- and postexercise assessment, to determine the efficacy of the exercise program and as a means of assessing the rate of progression of the program.

The intensity of the exercise should be such that pain, or discomfort, is experienced in the last set of 10 repetitions. This discomfort indicates that slight overloading of the tendon is occurring, which is necessary to increase its strength. We have observed that no pain indicates insufficient loading, and so no improvement in symptoms occurs. However, extreme pain, especially throughout the entire 30 repetitions, is a sign that too much force is being applied. This may act to worsen the patient's condition. *Incorrect evaluation of the level of pain or discomfort is the major cause of program failure.*

Table 3-1. Classification system for the
effect of pain on athletic performance

Level	Description of pain	Level of sports performance
1	No pain	Normal
2	Pain only with extreme exertion	Normal
3	Pain with extreme exertion and 1 to 2 hours afterward	Normal or slightly decreased
4	Pain during and after any vigorous activities	Somewhat decreased
5	Pain during activity and forcing termination	Markedly decreased
6	Pain during daily activities	Unable to perform

3. Exercise and the muscle-tendon unit

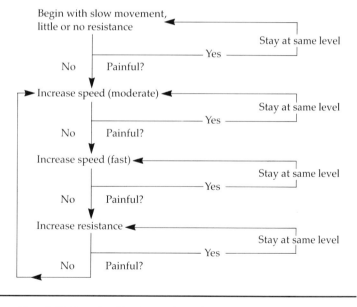

Figure 3-10. General outline of eccentric exercise program.

As the strength of the connective tissue increases, the pain will decrease and the force on the tendon can be increased until the pain recurs. This force increase is achieved by gradually increasing the speed of contraction from days 1 to 7.

In our experience, patients generally follow the progression outline in Figure 3-10.

Controlling the inflammation

Microstructural damage to the collagen fibers and disruption of the tendon microvasculature results in inflammation, which is heralded by pain. We have already discussed the deleterious effects of inflammation on the tendon (see Chapter 2) and the importance of controlling the inflammatory response. The application of ice immediately after trauma minimizes chemical activity and reduces pain. For these reasons, we recommend that ice be applied at the end of each treatment session and at more frequent intervals during treatment of acute tendinitis. Other measures, such as drugs or physical modalities, are left to the discretion of the individual physician or therapist. We have found them rarely necessary.

Summary

In this chapter we discuss the different types of muscle contraction and the effects of each in terms of force production. Although there is a paucity of experimental data dealing with the behavior of muscle during lengthening contractions as compared with the volume that exists concerning shortening contractions, results indicate that force increases with length for both eccentric and concentric contractions. The relationship between force and velocity differs, with force increasing with velocity of muscle contraction during eccentric exercise but decreasing as velocity increases during concentric exercise. The literature also suggests that eccentric contraction is a means by which muscles can maximize their force production while minimiz-

3. Exercise and the muscle-tendon unit

ing time delays and energy expenditure. Using this information and our clinical experience, we developed an exercise program to treat tendinitis. Pain, the cardinal sign of tendinitis, is used as both a classification of tendinitis severity and a yardstick of treatment progress.

3. Exercise and the muscle-tendon unit

4. *Achilles tendinitis*

All running athletes, including anyone who participates in a sport that involves running and jumping, risk incurring Achilles tendinitis. Since the fitness explosion and the development of jogging into a common recreational pastime and keep-fit method, more people have been exposed to the risk of Achilles tendinitis than ever before. In fact, Achilles tendinitis has become by far the most common athletic injury (Clancy 1982).

Like other tendinitides, Achilles tendinitis is difficult to treat, proving frustrating for both patient and therapist. This frustration has bred a plethora of treatment regimens, all of which meet with varying success at resolving the tendinitis.

In this chapter we review some of these regimens, along with the mechanics of Achilles tendinitis and the structure of the Achilles tendon. We also adapt the eccentric exercise program outlined in Chapter 3 to this specific athletic injury problem.

Structure of the Achilles tendon

The Achilles tendon is the common tendon of the gastrocnemius and soleus muscles. These two muscles are often referred to as the calf muscles, or triceps surae. The gastrocnemius arises from the lateral and medial femoral condyles, to which it is connected by strong, flat tendons. The soleus originates from the posterior surfaces of the tibia and fibula and lies beneath the gastrocnemius (see Fig. 4-1). The individual tendons of the gastrocnemius and soleus combine distally to form the Achilles tendon. Because of this arrangement, the Achilles tendon receives muscle fiber attachment from the soleus until just a few centimeters above its insertion onto the calcaneus. Note that the soleus and gastrocnemius contribute separately

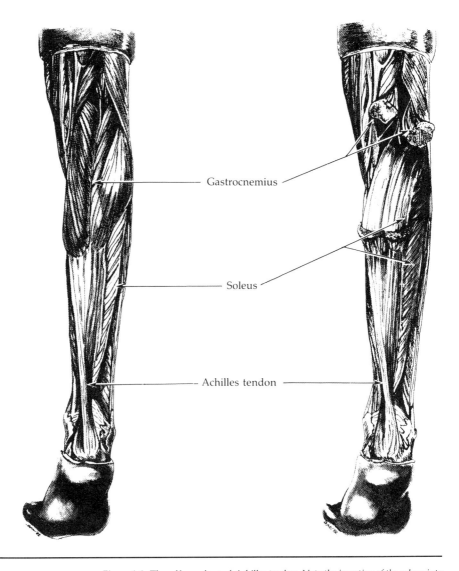

Gastrocnemius

Soleus

Achilles tendon

Figure 4-1. The calf muscles and Achilles tendon. Note the insertion of the soleus into the tendon until quite far down and the twist in the tendon as it descends.

to the formation of the Achilles tendon, and this contribution varies among individuals. The gastrocnemius portion varies from 26 to 11 cm in length. In comparison, the soleus contribution varies from 11 to 3 cm.

The Achilles tendon, initially fan-shaped and somewhat flattened near the gastrocnemius, becomes more rounded as it approaches the calcaneus, where it expands slightly to attach to its posterior surface. As it expands, the tendon gradually converts to fibrocartilage and stiffens as a result. Barfred (1971) postulates that this stiffness protects the tendon from oblique traction, just as the stiff cuff fitted on a flex close to an electric iron prevents buckling of the flex.

A second feature of note is that the tendon twists as it descends. The gastrocnemius portion usually makes up the more lateral and posterior portion of the tendon. As a whole, the tendon appears to rotate laterally as it descends. This rotation begins approximately 12 to 15 cm above the insertion and where the soleus begins to contribute fibers to the tendon. The degree of rotation depends on the amount of fusion between the gastrocnemius and soleus portions of the tendon. These two muscles may be separate through nearly their entire length or fused, depending on the individual. Minimal rotation seems to be associated with lengthy fusion.

Cummins et al. (1946) examined 100 tendons and described three patterns of rotation: type I, where the gastrocnemius contributes two-thirds of the posterior part of the tendon and the soleus contributes one-third; type II, where the gastrocnemius and soleus each contribute one-half; and type III, where the soleus makes up two-thirds of the posterior part of the tendon and the gastrocnemius makes up the other one-third. Type I is most common (52%), followed by type II (35%) and type III (13%).

This twisting produces areas of stress concentration in the tendon, caused by a "sawing" action of one part of the tendon on the other (Barfred 1971). This effect is most marked in the area 2 to 5 cm above

4. Achilles tendinitis

the tendon insertion where rotation is most pronounced. Interestingly, this is also the portion of the tendon with the poorest blood supply (Lagergren and Lindholm 1958) and the most common site of tendinitis.

The insertion of the Achilles tendon into the calcaneus is protected by two synovial bursae—the *subcutaneous* bursa between the skin and the tendon and the *retrocalcaneal* bursa between the tendon and the upper part of the calcaneus (see Fig. 4-2). Inflammation of either of these bursae (bursitis) may mimic the signs and symptoms of Achilles tendinitis.

Like other tendons, the Achilles tendon is composed of the familiar fibers, primary fiber bundles, and fascicles. The tendon is surrounded by a fine sheath called the epitenon. This sheath continues into the interior of the tendon, as the endotenon, to surround the primary and secondary fiber bundles (fascicles). The endotenon contains the internal vasculature of the tendon derived mainly from a bed of vessels in the mesotendon lying just beneath the tendon. This bed of vessels is an anastomosis from larger blood vessels in the area.

Covering the epitenon is a filmy layer of areolar tissue, the paratenon, which contains blood vessels running in a circular pattern around the epitenon. It acts as an elastic sleeve, allowing the tendon to move freely against, yet in continuity with, the surrounding tissue. The epitenon and paratenon together are often referred to as the *peritendon* (see Fig. 4-3).

Vascular supply   The Achilles tendon receives its blood supply at three locations: the musculotendinous junction, the tendon-bone junction, and along its length. The blood supply derived along the length of the tendon from the underlying mesotendon is most important. Small blood vessels arise from branches of the posterior tibial and peroneal arter-

---

4. Achilles tendinitis

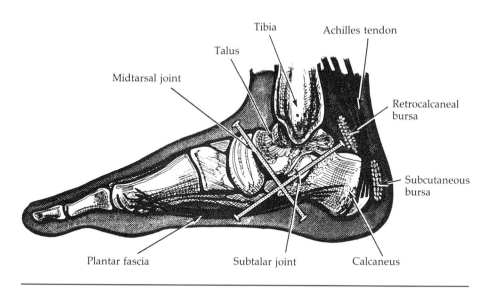

Figure 4-2. Bursae around the Achilles tendon.

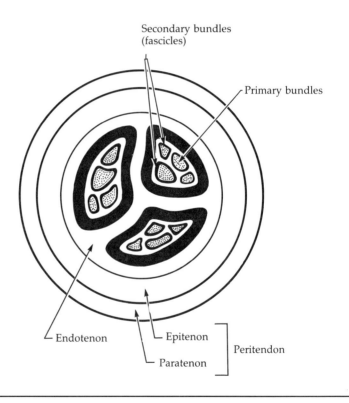

Figure 4-3. Layers of sheaths surrounding the Achilles tendon.

ies and anastomose in the mesotendon. From there they assume a course parallel with the longitudinal axis of the tendon in the endotenon.

Studies have shown that the vascularity of the Achilles tendon is reduced 2 to 6 cm above its insertion (Inglis et al. 1976; Lea and Smith 1972), a site that appears common for rupture (Lindholm and Arner 1959). The association between a zone of reduced vascularity and tendon rupture was shown by Rathbun and MacNab (1970) in their study of the supraspinatus tendon at the shoulder joint. The presence of such a zone in the Achilles tendon is considered to play an etiologic role in ruptures of that tendon (Smart, Taunton, and Clement 1980).

Although the reason for reduced vascularity in the supraspinatus tendon was linked to pressure from the overlying acromion, no such cause has been demonstrated in the Achilles tendon. Perhaps the area of reduced vascularity coincides with the cessation of insertion of the soleus muscle fibers into the tendon; or twisting may compromise the microvasculature when the tendon is under tension.

Classification of Achilles tendon disease

It is difficult to classify Achilles tendon disorders because of the possibilities of different types. For example, many authors distinguish between a "true" tendinitis and tenosynovitis. The term *tenosynovitis*, however, does not strictly apply in the case of the Achilles tendon, since it is covered by a peritendon, not a synovial sheath. Recognizing this, some authors (Puddu et al. 1976; Smart, Taunton, and Clement 1980) prefer the term *peritendinitis*. They propose a classification of tendinosis and peritendinitis, with the former indicating disruption of the actual tendon and the latter being inflammation of the tendon sheath. This definition can extend also to combinations of tendinosis and peritendinitis and partial rupture.

---

4. Achilles tendinitis

Undoubtedly there are cases in which symptoms are due primarily to inflammation of the tendon sheath, that is, peritendinitis. But the number of these cases that do *not* involve injury to the tendon as well must be very small. Since the injury may be at the microscopic level, subsequent inflammation can take place without visible change in the tendon. Sometimes symptoms can be precipitated through pressure on the tendon, such as from a high heel counter on a running shoe or a tightly laced skate, and cause irritation of the peritendon alone. More commonly, either the retrocalcaneal or subcutaneous bursa is involved.

Most symptomatic cases of Achilles tendinitis involve trauma to the actual Achilles tendon, as described in Chapter 2. The injury may be on a fibrillar level or greater. The resulting inflammatory response causes pain, which increases with the magnitude of the injury. As a result, we prefer to use the classification system outlined in Chapter 3 (see Table 3-1, p. 64). Injuries that cannot be classified by this system are usually easy to diagnose since they are caused by an external force, such as a blow or pressure from footwear. Although not initially considered "true" tendinitis, the inflammatory changes accompanying these injuries may cause weakening of the tendon and predispose it to tendinitis.

Etiology

Mechanics

Tendons are adapted to withstand tensile forces, and their fibers are aligned in response to this type of force. In areas where tendons must withstand or "absorb" large forces, they are usually found to be long in relation to their accompanying muscles because the tendon is much stronger than the muscle per unit area. Long tendons are also able to "store" some of this force for brief periods and use it to perform movement, much as a stretched elastic band assists movement when it is released (Murray et al. 1978). (This is the concept of elastic energy, which is discussed in Chapter 3.)

---

4. Achilles tendinitis

At first glance, the Achilles tendon seems well suited to withstand the external forces encountered in walking and running since generally its fibers are longitudinally oriented. However, recall that the tendon twists as it descends, producing areas of stress concentration as one part of the tendon saws across another. This sawlike action is compounded by the fact that the tendon is not homogeneous, but receives interdigitating fibers from the soleus.

The ankle is a hinge joint with motion in one plane only (sagittal) which leads to the assumption that any force applied to the Achilles tendon produces motion only about an axis through the ankle joint. This apparent simplicity is contradicted when we consider that motion at the subtalar joint also affects (and is affected by) the Achilles tendon. Motion at the subtalar joint occurs in the frontal and transverse planes, producing inversion-eversion and abduction-adduction movements, respectively. Movement in the transverse plane twists and untwists the Achilles tendon. Inversion and eversion place unequal tensile forces on different parts of the tendon which can result in a bowstring effect in the Achilles tendon (Smart, Taunton, and Clement 1980). Barfred (1971) emphasizes the fact that all tendons passing one or more joints with axes of movement at right angles to each other may be exposed to oblique traction. A 30° change in the position of the hindfoot, he notes, results in one side of the tendon being elongated 10 percent more than fibers on the other side. However, these movements are necessary to allow accommodation of the foot to uneven ground.

Various authors (Alexander and Vernon 1975b; Ljungqvist 1968; Smith 1975) have estimated the force in the Achilles tendon during such activities as walking, running, and landing from a jump. These forces range from approximately 1962 to 2354 N in walking to between 3924 and 5886 N in running and up to 8729 N in fast running. The stress on the tendon (force per unit area) can be calculated by dividing these values by the tendon's cross-sectional area. The maximum value of stress for the mammalian tendon is estimated to be

4. Achilles tendinitis

49 to 98 MPa (Elliott 1965). Table 4-1 shows the stresses on the Achilles tendon during various activities based on a theoretical cross-sectional area of 75 mm^2.

Stresses applied to the Achilles tendon during athletic activities, however, appear to exceed these maximum levels. Unfortunately, the most accurate information available on tendon behavior during activities such as walking and running comes from animal studies, where forces and strains can be measured directly. Data on human tendons have been derived from laboratory studies or estimated from film and force platform data. It is difficult to make direct comparisons between stresses estimated during activities and those determined under laboratory conditions, because the latter are derived from tests performed on isolated tendon specimens which are elongated at a constant rate until failure. Under these controlled conditions, the strain rates may be considerably lower than those that take place during activities, which alters the load that the tendon is able to bear (Kear and Smith 1975; Lochner et al. 1980). Thus the maximum tendon stress value of 49 to 98 MPa may be lower than that which occurs at higher strain rates and may be lower than the actual maximum strength of the tendon. The superposition of factors such as heel varus or valgus, tibial torsion, or excessive tightness in the calf muscles may also lead to areas of stress concentration in the tendon, increasing the likelihood of microtears (see Fig. 4-4).

Table 4-1. Stress in Achilles tendon with different activities

Activity	Area (mm^2)	Force (N)	Stress (MPa)
Walking	75	1962–2354	26.1–31.4
Running, slow	75	3924–5886	52.3–78.5
Running, fast	75	8729	117.7
Jumping	75	1962	26.1

4. Achilles tendinitis

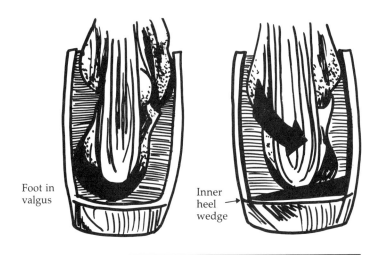

Foot in
valgus

Inner
heel
wedge

Figure 4-4. A valgus hindfoot stretches the inner part of the tendon more. This is readily corrected with a small medial heel wedge.

Role of eccentric contraction

Ljungqvist (1968), in a review of 92 cases of partial Achilles tendon rupture, lists the following situations as most likely to cause injury to the Achilles tendon:

1. Pushing off with the weight-bearing foot while simultaneously extending the knee, common in sprinting or running uphill. The calf muscles are maximally contracted.
2. Sudden and unexpected dorsiflexion of the ankle, such as slipping on a stair or stumbling into a hole, where the heel drops suddenly. The calf muscles are moderately contracted but become maximally contracted in reflex to the sudden stretch.
3. Violent dorsiflexion while the foot is plantarflexed, such as in jumping and falling. The calf muscles are maximally contracted, and sudden movement leads to marked stretching of the muscle and particularly the tendon.

All these examples involve eccentric contraction of the muscle; that is, the muscle is contracting and lengthening as the tendon is stretched. Athletes suffering from Achilles tendinitis characteristically feel more pain during an eccentric movement and can frequently recall specific motions, much like those mentioned, that are painful.

There appears to be a contradiction between the fact that isolated tendon specimens are stronger when tested at higher strain rates and the clinical impression that sudden movement appears more likely to injure the tendon. On the basis of experimental findings, one would expect the tendon to increase its resistance to injury as it is stretched more rapidly. This cannot be readily explained, except to say that extremely rapid movements do not allow time for protective measures, such as relaxing the muscle, to occur. The stresses on the tendon with differing strain rates have not been investigated experimentally, nor are the normally occurring strain rates known. Thus, more research is needed before the exact nature of the interaction between rates of loading and strain can be understood.

---

4. Achilles tendinitis

Footwear

Footwear may contribute to Achilles tendinitis in a number of ways. Loose heel counters and narrow heels may not afford sufficient stability to the subtalar joint. A high, poorly padded heel counter may cause undue pressure on the tendon.

Inadequate heel elevation also may be a factor. Flat shoes may cause the tendon to be stretched farther at heel strike. Since most walking shoes have heels, switching to flat shoes may overstretch the shortened tendon. This effect suggests that athletes who use flat shoes (such as tennis players or basketball players) may be particularly vulnerable to Achilles tendinitis. Yet runners are more likely to suffer it because of the many more times that the tendon is loaded—each time the foot strikes the ground.

To lessen the propensity for Achilles tendinitis, the shoe sole should be flexible and soft enough to cushion heel impact during running. A rigid sole increases the distance from the ankle at which the force must be applied during push-off (moment arm), thus increasing the ankle joint moment. This moment is "balanced" by one in the opposite direction created by the force of the calf muscles acting through the Achilles tendon. The mathematical product of this force and the perpendicular distance (moment arm) between the tendon and the ankle joint center equals the magnitude of this moment. Thus, as the joint moment increases, so does the force in the tendon. Shoes should be examined to ensure that they bend readily in the forefoot at a level corresponding to the metatarsal-phalangeal joints.

Training

Sudden alterations in style or quantity of training can produce microtrauma in the Achilles tendon. Certain changes are particularly likely to precipitate tendinitis:

1. Changing shoes
2. Adding hills or sprints to regular training

4. Achilles tendinitis

3. Running on uneven ground
4. Changing running surface (as when ground freezes)
5. Inadequate emphasis on warm-up and flexibility
6. Beginning another sport such as basketball, tennis, or squash
7. Sudden increase in mileage
8. Resumption of training after a long period of inactivity

Examination

Case history

The importance of the case history cannot be overemphasized. Since pain is the usual symptom that causes the athlete to seek help, the examiner must determine *where* the pain is, *when* it occurs, *how long* it lasts, and the time elapsed since symptoms were first noticed. The duration of pain and its severity are particularly important in classifying the degree of tendinitis. Questions concerning other causative factors such as training changes also should be included in the initial workup. This will help reveal whether any training factors are implicated in causing the tendinitis. Careful examination of the running shoe and the foot in both standing and non-weight-bearing situations is mandatory for physicians and trainers attempting to isolate a cause for the presenting tendinitis. This will enable the examiner to see whether structural or alignment problems are contributing to the problem.

Clinical examination

The injured tendon should be palpated along its length in both the relaxed (plantarflexed) and taut (dorsiflexed) positions and compared with the contralateral side. This is best done with the patient lying prone. Swelling of the paratenon, unlike thickening of the tendon tissue, is superficial and feels less "solid." Pressure on the swollen segment often produces pain. Not infrequently, a thickened area will be noted. This may indicate a previous injury to the tendon or areas of focal degeneration.

4. Achilles tendinitis

Examination of joint range and muscle tightness should be performed also. A quick check can readily be done by having the athlete lean forward against a support with the heel on the floor and the knee straight. Ask the patient to bend the knee of the extended leg. The bent knee should allow more dorsiflexion because the gastrocnemius is partially relaxed. If dorsiflexion does not increase, then tightness of the soleus muscle is present.

Finally, functional tests such as hopping on one foot or dropping the heel rapidly over the edge of a step may be used to determine whether eccentric contraction of the calf muscles is involved in the injury. These tests frequently produce pain on landing during hopping or pain at the end of the range of movement in dropping over a support, and are important in a complete assessment of the problem.

Other possible disorders confused with Achilles tendinitis

Achilles tendinitis may be confused with other athletic injuries, including some of the following:

1. Bone bruises
   a. Caused by a direct blow to the calcaneus, usually at the plantar surface.
   b. Relieved by removing pressure on the painful area.
2. Bursitis
   a. Either retrocalcaneal or subcutaneous.
   b. Usually related to external pressure from shoe or skate.
3. Plantar fasciitis
   a. Inflammation of calcaneal attachment of plantar fascia.
   b. Characterized by tenderness at the point of insertion and sharp pain during weight-bearing activities, especially during push-off.
   c. Etiology is varied; may be weak foot intrinsic muscles, overweight, flat foot, and so on.
   d. Symptomatic relief most easily obtained with orthotics.
   e. Physiotherapy or anti-inflammatory drugs may be useful.

---

4. *Achilles tendinitis*

4. Fracture
   a. A stress fracture may result from repetitive trauma or from same factors that cause tendinitis.
   b. Pain increases with intensity and is felt at rest.
   c. Activity is usually impossible.
5. Muscle tear
   a. Usually related to a single traumatic episode.
   b. Accompanied by swelling, bruising, and pain.
6. Posterior tibial tendinitis (shin splints)
   a. Pain along medial border of tibia.
   b. Causes much the same as for Achilles tendinitis.
   c. Often faulty foot alignment is involved; best solved with use of orthotics.
7. Compartment syndrome
   a. Pain in lower leg related to increased pressure in one of fascial compartments of leg.
   b. Requires careful evaluation and possibly surgery.

Treatment

Conservative treatment, as outlined in Chapter 2, is generally used to deal with Achilles tendinitis. Modalities include rest, anti-inflammatory drugs, ultrasound, orthotics, cast immobilization, and so on. When these methods fail, as they frequently do, sometimes surgery is performed. Although these treatments may relieve symptoms, recurrence is common because the basic cause of the problem is not being dealt with—an Achilles tendon too weak to do what is demanded of it. There is sufficient current (and some past) evidence to show that inactivity actually weakens the tendon structure. Thus, while rest or surgery (which is inevitably followed by rest) may succeed in relieving symptoms in some cases, these are not the treatments of choice. A vicious cycle begins, with rest weakening the tendon so that symptoms recur as soon as activity is resumed. Eventually any vigorous physical activity provokes symptoms. Only in cases of acute tendinitis, where pain is so intense as to prevent athletic participation, should complete rest be enforced and then only

---

4. Achilles tendinitis

until the acute symptoms subside. Anti-inflammatory drugs may be helpful during this period.

The use of corticosteroid injections in treating Achilles tendinitis is strongly discouraged. Kennedy and Baxter-Willis (1976) have shown that physiologic doses of steroid placed directly into the normal tendon weaken it significantly for up to 14 days after injection. The incidence of tendon rupture after steroid injection is also very high (Ljungqvist 1968).

The eccentric program

The program of exercise outlined in Chapter 3 can be applied to Achilles tendinitis also. The first step is a *warm-up,* followed by *flexibility* exercises for the calf muscles (see Fig. 4-5). The warm-up may consist of any moderately vigorous activity such as sit-ups, push-ups, and so forth.

Next, three sets of 10 repetitions of the eccentric exercise are carried out. This is most easily done by having the patient stand on the edge of a step. The body weight is supported on the ball of the foot, so the heel is free. Then allow the heel to drop downward with gravity, below the level of the step (see Fig. 4-6).

Progression is made by increasing the speed of movement or increasing the resistance. The program proceeds as follows:

1. Weight is supported equally on both feet throughout the exercise session.
2. Increase shifting of weight to symptomatic leg.
3. Weight is supported on symptomatic leg only.
4. Increase speed of dropping.
5. Add weight to shoulders.

The severity of the initial symptoms determines the starting resistance. The indication for an increase in resistance is the absence of

4. Achilles tendinitis

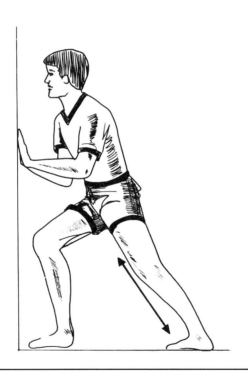

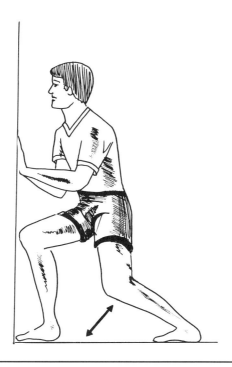

Figure 4-5. Stretching the gastrocnemius (left) *and soleus* (right) *muscles.*

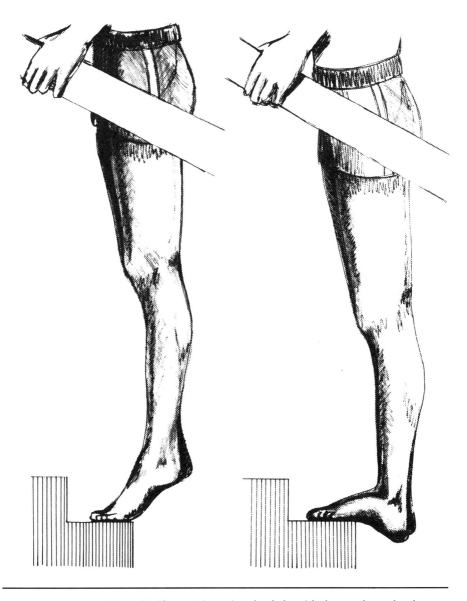

Figure 4-6. The eccentric exercise—drop body weight downward over edge of support.

Table 4-2. Eccentric exercise program for Achilles tendinitis

Week	Days	Exercise	Activity level
1	1 to 3	Slow drop, bilateral weight support	Cannot participate
	3 to 5	Moderate speed, bilateral support	
	6, 7	Fast drop, bilateral support	
2	1 to 3	Slow, increased weight on symptomatic leg	Cannot participate in sports
	3 to 5	Moderate, increased weight	
	6, 7	Fast, increased weight	
3	1 to 3	Slow, weight supported on symptomatic leg	Pain during rapid drop; active in sports, but limited
	3 to 5	Moderate, weight on one leg	
	6, 7	Fast speed	
4	1 to 3	Slow, add 10% of body weight	Pain during vigorous activity
	3 to 5	Moderate, same weight	
	6, 7	Fast speed	
5	1 to 3	Slow, increase by 5 to 10 lb	Pain only during exertion
	3 to 5	Moderate speed	
	6, 7	Fast speed	
6	1 to 3	Slow, increase 5 to 10 lb	Rarely experience pain
	3 to 5	Moderate speed	
	6, 7	Fast speed	

4. Achilles tendinitis

pain at the end of 30 repetitions. For example, an athlete whose symptoms were present during any activity, such as running on level ground, and who experienced pain when dropping over the edge of the step would start at *slow* speed with body weight supported on *both* feet. An athlete who experiences pain only during extreme exertion, such as sprinting uphill, may start the program with weight placed on the shoulders and supported on one leg. Generally, adding 10 percent of body weight is a suitable starting point for this phase of the program, although trial and error may change that rule. The summary of progression is shown in Table 4-2, which includes suggested starting points based on the level of symptoms.

Since each athlete varies in body weight and size and in the severity of symptoms experienced, we recommend the program be monitored by the amount of discomfort the patient experiences. There should be some discomfort in the last 10 of the 30 repetitions, but pain should *not* be present throughout and the level of pain should not be extreme. Ignoring pain, the body's warning signal, means further damage may occur. Progression should not take place until discomfort is absent or minimal.

Often there will be little or no change in symptoms during the first 2 or 3 weeks of the program. Indeed, patients may experience a slight increase in the pain felt during athletic activity. This is normal but can be very discouraging to the athlete who will need to be reassured that he or she must continue the program.

The question most often asked during this time is, When will the symptoms disappear? This is related to the severity of symptoms when the program began and the prior duration of symptoms. In an athlete who experiences pain only infrequently with maximum exertion, symptoms should be alleviated within 6 weeks. Individuals with more severe symptoms that have been present for a longer time may only begin to see improvement in 6 weeks, and complete relief may take considerably longer.

---

4. Achilles tendinitis

5. Jumper's knee

The jumping athlete subjects the patellar tendon to tremendous forces with each explosive jumping movement. Repetition of such movements can cause trauma to the tendon, producing patellar tendinitis, or "jumper's knee." Basketball and volleyball players are especially vulnerable to this disorder because of the high demands placed on their quadriceps. However, athletes involved in running, cycling, kicking, or other jumping events may be similarly afflicted.

Although many case reports in the literature discuss patellar tendon rupture, only a few studies deal with patellar tendinitis (Blazina 1973; Martens et al. 1982), and the information on treatment is sparse. Also, symptoms may be easily mistaken for those of other common knee disorders such as patellofemoral arthroses.

In this chapter, we review the structure and mechanics of the knee extensor mechanism, the etiology and differential diagnosis of jumper's knee, and the treatment of this disorder. Again, activity in the form of eccentric exercise is stressed.

Structure and function

The quadriceps femoris covers most of the front and sides of the femur and is the great extensor muscle of the leg. It is divided into four parts, hence its name. The rectus femoris and vastus intermedius, the most central portions of the muscle, jointly form the quadriceps tendon (see Fig. 5-1). The vastus lateralis, the largest part of the quadriceps, contracts into a flat tendon attached to the lateral border of the patella and the quadriceps tendon. The vastus medialis has a broad, aponeurotic attachment to the medial border of the patella and the quadriceps tendon. Its lower fibers, almost horizontally oriented, form the characteristic bulge seen just medial to the patella when the extensor muscles are contracted. The patella lies

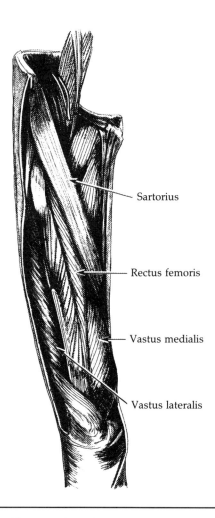

Sartorius

Rectus femoris

Vastus medialis

Vastus lateralis

Figure 5-1. The quadriceps muscle (vastus intermedius not shown).

within the quadriceps and provides protection for the knee joint. It also increases the length of the moment arm of the quadriceps, an action frequently described as "increasing the mechanical advantage of the muscle."

The tendons of the different portions of the quadriceps unite in the lower thigh to form a single strong tendon attached to the base of the patella. The fibers of this quadriceps tendon enclose the patella and pass over it to blend with the ligamentum patellae, or patellar tendon, which inserts on the tibial tubercle.

There is some debate as to the description of the infrapatellar portion of the quadriceps tendon. Most people consider it a continuation of the tendon of the muscle and thus call it the patellar tendon. Others claim it differs from ordinary tendons and is closer to a ligament in structure. Since the ultrastructure and biochemistry of the tendon have not been well studied, this question remains open. We use the term *patellar tendon* in our discussion.

Essentially the ultrastructure of the patellar tendon follows the description in Chapter 1. Like other tendons, it is stiffer and more avascular near its bony attachments. The reduced blood supply in these areas makes them slow to heal and prone to chronic tendinitis. Thus we expect the attachments to the patella and the tibial tubercle to be the most common sites of tendinitis; and, indeed, this is so.

Sites of patellar tendinitis

There are three possible locations for patellar tendinitis: (1) at the insertion on the tibial tubercle, (2) at the inferior pole of the patella, and (3) at the base of the patella. Interestingly, the vulnerability of these locations to tendinitis is age-specific. The first is more common in growing children or adolescents, and the last in athletes over 40 years of age.

---

5. *Jumper's knee*

Insertion on tibial tubercle

In growing children, the tibial tubercle is part of the upper epiphysis of the tibia and is the "weak link" in the extensor mechanism. The traction of the tendon on the tubercle elevates it from the tibial shaft, forming the characteristic bump of what is often referred to as Osgood-Schlatter disease.

Inferior pole of the patella

This is true patellar tendinitis, and it occurs at the attachment of the tendon to the inferior pole of the patella. It is by far the most common site of the patellar tendinitides, and usually it is seen in individuals between late adolescence and 40 years of age. In fact, 80 percent of cases of patellar tendinitis in this age group are located at this site. Occasionally this type of tendinitis occurs in younger age groups and is called Sinding-Larsen-Johansson disease. In these cases, however, a separate area of calcification is present in the patellar tendon (Medlar and Lyne 1978). Thus it appears very similar in etiology to Osgood-Schlatter disease.

The etiologic factor in adult patellar tendinitis seems to be the concentration of stress that occurs at this site owing to the narrowing of the tendon. The stress increases with knee flexion and can lead to tendinitis.

Base of the patella

Despite the term *base*, we actually are referring to the most proximal portion of the patella. This is the most common site of tendinitis in people over age 40. Yet overall patellar tendinitis occurs relatively infrequently in athletes in this age group. The reason is unclear, but we may speculate that the increasing stiffness of the tendon renders it more resistant to injury as the person ages.

---

5. Jumper's knee

The signs, symptoms, and functional disabilities are similar for all three kinds of patellar tendinitis; so is the treatment. Yet recognition of these locations is important in differential diagnosis, as we see later in this chapter. (See Fig. 5-2.)

The lesion

Patellar tendinitis is a chronic overload lesion in the tendon. Excessive stress in this part of the tendon during repetitive movement of the extensor mechanism of the knee results in microtearing within the tendon, followed by fraying of the tendon fibers and focal degeneration. As a useful analogy, consider a rope after some of its woven fibers have been ruptured. The ends of these fibers fray, and more stress is placed on the remaining fibers, so that they may eventually fail as well.

The lesion in patellar tendinitis is usually situated in the deep fibers of the tendon near its insertion. There are two reasons for this. First, the fibers near the center of the tendon exhibit less crimping and so are less elastic. Second, bending of the fibers with knee flexion occurs at a more acute angle near the center of the tendon. Anatomic examination (Martens et al. 1982) revealed consistent findings of mucoid degeneration and fibrinoid necrosis within the tendon. The inflammatory response to injury causes pain and weakens the remaining fibers, predisposing the tendon to further injury. Thus patellar tendinitis is usually chronic and progressive since the same loads are being applied to an increasingly weaker structure.

In healthy individuals, the patella is considered the weakest link in the extensor mechanism by some authors (Miskew, Pearson, and Pankovich 1980). This means that violent quadriceps contraction on a flexed knee will cause a transverse fracture of the patella across the fulcrum of the femoral condyles. Contractions are rarely this violent, however, and microtrauma rather than macrotrauma occurs. This trauma will affect the tendon if any degenerative changes are present, since then it becomes the weakest link in the system. We also

5. Jumper's knee

95

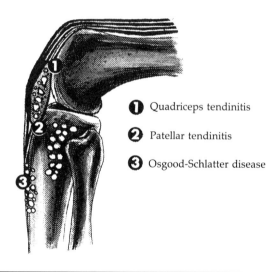

1. Quadriceps tendinitis

2. Patellar tendinitis

3. Osgood-Schlatter disease

Figure 5-2. Three common sites of patellar tendinitis (jumper's knee).

believe there are very few athletes who have not suffered some degenerative changes in their tendon simply owing to their sports involvement. Usually these are minor in nature, and the athlete is asymptomatic.

Signs and
symptoms

Pain

As usual, pain is the predominant symptom and the one that causes the athlete to seek assistance. The pain is usually very localized, so careful questioning about the exact site of pain (and having the person point out the painful spot) should be very helpful. You should note *when* the pain is felt and *how long* it lasts, since these facts indicate the severity of the injury. The role of eccentric contraction should be ascertained also. We have found that most athletes experience greater pain when landing from a jump or immediately prior to takeoff following the eccentric preparatory phase. (See Fig. 5-3.)

Tenderness

Palpation of the likely painful site, as determined by the patient's age and description, often reveals tenderness. This sign confirms the diagnosis of patellar tendinitis.

Inflammation

Pain is a result of inflammation. Sometimes it is possible to palpate increased temperature and some soft-tissue swelling. These signs are uncommon, however, and usually appear in long-standing cases in which nearby soft tissues, such as the infrapatellar fat pad, are also irritated.

Stiffness

Patients commonly complain of stiffness if they keep the knee in one position for any length of time and particularly if that position is knee flexion, such as that required by sitting in a car or at a movie.

---

5. Jumper's knee

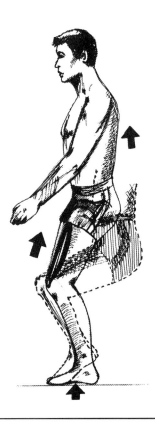

Figure 5-3. The largest forces occur during the eccentric phase of landing from a jump.

The patient with Osgood-Schlatter disease may demonstrate an enlarged tibial tubercle. Usually this is found in the older adolescent who has had symptoms for a long time or who has stopped growing. Another sign is a decline in athletic performance, such as decreased vertical jumping ability. One very helpful sign is the occurrence of pain following a rapid eccentric force applied to the extended leg. This is easily done by applying manual pressure to the limb, as shown in Figure 5-4.

Classification
Blazina (1973) proposed the first classification of patellar tendon disorder (see Table 5-1). We prefer to use the classification described in Chapters 3 and 4 and shown again in Table 5-2.

Etiology
A discussion of the etiology of patellar tendinitis requires consideration of the forces applied to the tendon during various activities. (These are summarized in Table 5-3.) There is considerable variation in some of these forces, but large stresses that nearly match the maximum tensile strength of the tendon can take place in normal athletic activities such as running.

A few studies provide particularly valuable insight into the role of eccentric movement in patellar tendinitis. Wahrenberg, Lindbeck, and Ekholm (1978) recorded the tendon tension force and EMG activity during the kicking of a soccer ball and found that the maximum tension occurred very early in the movement, when the initial knee flexion changed to extension, long before the ball was hit. This coincided with the peak of quadriceps EMG activity. This study points out that a force of 5200 N, the highest value obtained, corresponds to 7 times body weight and that this tensile force is generated in a freely moving limb. Repetition of such forces may result in tendinitis.

5. Jumper's knee

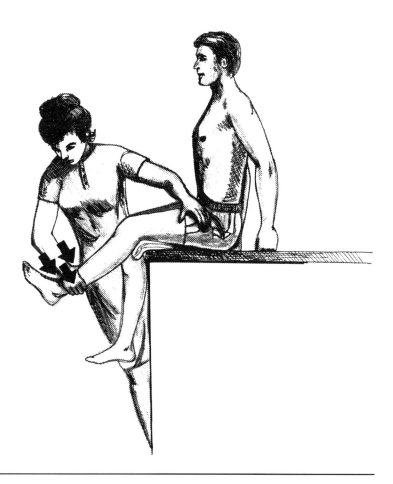

Figure 5-4. Have the patient extend the leg, then suddenly *apply downward pressure. This may reproduce the symptoms.*

Table 5-1. Classification of patellar disorder according to Blazina

Stage 1	Pain only after sports activity
Stage 2	Pain at the beginning of sports activity disappearing after warm-up and reappearing with fatigue
Stage 3	Constant pain at rest and during activity; patient unable to participate in sports at previous level
Stage 4	Complete rupture of patellar tendon

Table 5-2. Classification of patellar disorder according to pain

Level 1	No pain
Level 2	Pain with extreme exertion only; does not hinder sports performance and disappears when activity stops
Level 3	Pain with exertion, remains 1 to 2 hours afterward
Level 4	Pain during any athletic activity, lasts 4 to 6 hours afterward, increases throughout activity; performance level decreased
Level 5	Pain starts immediately after activity commences, causes withdrawal from activity
Level 6	Pain during daily activities; patient unable to participate in any sports

Table 5-3. Forces in patellar tendon during activities

Activity	Force (N)	Stress (MPa)
Running	7500–9000	37.5–45.0
Kicking	5200	26.0
Jumping (landing)	8000	40.0
Jumping (takeoff)	2500	12.5
Walking	500	2.5

5. Jumper's knee

In activities involving weight bearing, such as running and jumping, there is a potential for even greater forces, especially with rapid motions. Adding extra weight naturally increases the force. Zernicke, Garhammer, and Jobe (1977) were able to obtain data concerning the force that produced tendon rupture in a weight lifter. The athlete suffered a patellar tendon rupture during filming of a 175-kg lift. They estimated the patellar tendon tension at the time of rupture to be 14,500 N, or more than 17 times the lifter's body weight. Furthermore, the rupture took place at the peak in the knee joint moment that occurred as the lifter stopped the downward motion of his body and the weight. This article provides one of the few examples in which the magnitude of load and the loading rate have been estimated during an actual injury. Clearly human subjects cannot approach maximum loading conditions experimentally (see Fig. 5-5).

The magnitudes of these forces seem to indicate that the patellar tendon is frequently subjected to loads approaching maximum during athletic activities. In addition, these loads are repeated. This cyclic loading reduces the ability of the tendon to elongate because it is unable to restore its molecular structure (Krahl 1976). Thus the tendon, which is perfectly elastic only in the area of 3 to 4 percent elongation caused by loads of less than one-quarter maximum, may suffer microtears. It was previously thought (Elliott 1965) that tendons were probably not stressed to greater than one-quarter of their maximum tensile strength in vivo; however, more recent evidence suggests that near maximal forces are applied regularly.

We believe that eccentric movement is the major etiologic factor in patellar tendinitis, because of the higher patellar tendon tensions associated with eccentric contraction. This belief originates from patient statements describing maximum discomfort while landing from a jump or during rapid backward movement, as in tennis, and is supported by experimental evidence such as that of Wahrenberg, Lindbeck, and Ekholm (1978) and Zernicke, Garhammer, and Jobe (1977).

---

5. Jumper's knee

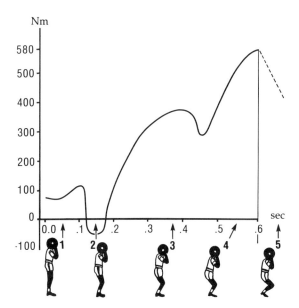

Mean resultant knee-joint moments from the
beginning of the jerk motion until 0.04 sec after
tendon failure.

*Figure 5-5. A knee-joint moment-time curve during a lift in which the patellar
tendon ruptured. Forces were estimated at greater than 17 times body weight when
the rupture occurred. Redrawn with permission from Zernicke, R.F., Garhammer,
J., Jobe, F.W., Human patellar-tendon rupture.* J. Bone Joint Surg. *59A(2):179–
183, 1977.*

Knee joint complaints are probably most common in athletes and can easily be confusing to the inexperienced examiner. A careful history usually allows you to make a tentative diagnosis which can be confirmed by physical examination. The following are some conditions that may be mistaken for patellar tendinitis.

Patellofemoral arthrosis

Patellofemoral arthrosis is easily confused with patellar tendinitis because of the similarity in symptoms—pain on squatting and jumping, stiffness after sitting, and so on. However, unlike tendinitis, there is no point tenderness at the usual sites of patellar tendinitis, nor is pain specific to eccentric activities. Quadriceps wasting is usually much more obvious in cases involving the patellofemoral joint.

Meniscal tear

The history of this injury is different from that of tendinitis. A rotational injury is involved in most meniscal lesions. Locking and joint effusion are characteristic, and tenderness is present along the joint line. None of these symptoms is present in jumper's knee.

Infrapatellar fat pad inflammation (Hoffa's disease)

The infrapatellar fat pad can be irritated through overuse or following direct pressure on the anterior infrapatellar aspect of the knee. The symptoms mimic those of patellofemoral arthrosis and patellar tendinitis, but usually can be distinguished by the presence of pain when the fat pad is gently squeezed between the fingers and thumb. Swelling of the fat pad may be evident also.

5. Jumper's knee

Bursitis

Of the numerous bursae around the knee, four are related to the quadriceps muscle (see Fig. 5-6):

1. *Suprapatellar bursa*—between the anterior surface of the lower femur and the deep surface of the quadriceps
2. *Subcutaneous prepatellar bursa*—between the lower part of the patella and the skin
3. *Subcutaneous infrapatellar bursa*—between the lower part of the tibial tuberosity and the skin
4. *Deep infrapatellar bursa*—between the patellar tendon and the tibia

Bursitis can be easily confused with patellar tendinitis, especially in the case of deep infrapatellar bursitis, since tension in the tendon will compress the bursa and cause pain. Tenderness with pressure on the tibial tubercle is present. Since this site is uncommon for tendinitis beyond the adolescent years, one can suspect bursitis in older patients.

Treatment

General

The treatment of patellar tendinitis, for most clinicians, is no less frustrating than that of Achilles tendinitis, and the same variety of methods have been developed.

Frequently, cast immobilization is used to afford a period of rest for the tendon. This usually follows other conservative treatment measures such as stretching exercises, ultrasound, deep-friction massage, knee supports, oral anti-inflammatory agents, and abstinence from sports. If a cast is applied, symptoms usually have disappeared by the time the cast is removed. Unfortunately they soon recur, since loads of the same magnitude are being applied to a tendon that has been weakened by immobility. Furthermore, quadri-

---

5. *Jumper's knee*

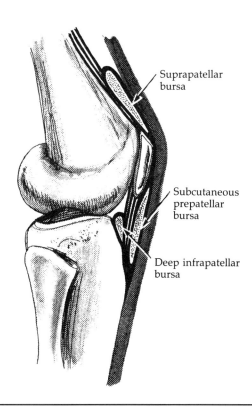

Figure 5-6. Bursae around the knee joint that may mimic patellar tendinitis.

ceps and calf muscle atrophy, and joint stiffness must be dealt with. The basic outline for the conservative treatment of patellar tendinitis is presented in Table 5-4, which follows Blazina's classification system.

The use of cast immobilization is decreasing as more people realize that it extends an already long period of immobility and gives only temporary relief of symptoms (Martens et al. 1982).

The use of steroid injections is also discouraged because of the danger of tendon rupture. Steroid injections provide temporary pain relief but cause mechanical damage to the tendon (see Chapter 2). In many studies of patients whose tendons rupture, a history of previous cortisone (steroid) injections has been noted. The absence of symptoms frequently causes the athlete to perform beyond his or her physical limits, thereby increasing the likelihood of further damage to the tendon.

Table 5-4. Conservative treatment program for patellar tendinitis[a]

Stage 1	Adequate warming up
	(5 to 10 minutes of push-ups, sit-ups, etc.)
	Ice after activity
	Local anti-inflammatory treatment and anti-inflammatory drugs for several weeks
	Physiotherapy, including isometric quadriceps exercises
	Elastic knee support
Stage 2	Same as stage 1
	Some form of heat before activity
	Period of rest
Stage 3	Same as stage 2 but also prolonged period of rest
	If conservative treatment fails, abstinence from sports or surgery
Stage 4	Primary repair of tendon

[a]Correlates with classification system in Table 5-1 (Blazina).

5. Jumper's knee

Surgery is also becoming less popular as a treatment method, except in cases of tendon rupture, where it is essential. Typically, surgery involves resection of the degenerated or necrotic tendon tissue, with or without drilling of the inferior pole of the patella to stimulate the growth of new blood vessels. This treatment is usually followed by a period of immobilization (4 to 6 weeks) and 3 to 8 months of rehabilitation. While some authors claim excellent results after surgical treatment (Blazina 1973; Martens et al. 1982), no controlled studies comparing a treatment *identical* with the one that follows surgery have been performed. It seems quite plausible that over a 4-month period of rest from sport considerable improvement in symptoms will occur.

The eccentric program

Despite the success or failure of other treatment methods, the fact remains that the tendon is damaged when its tensile strength is exceeded. Thus a treatment program to increase this tensile strength should make the tendon less susceptible to injury.

We agree with many of the conservative treatment methods, particularly the importance of warm-up and flexibility exercises before activity and ice application after. Flexibility training is important because not only does it increase the elasticity of the muscle-tendon unit, but also it may increase the tensile strength of the tendon.

However, the main advantage of the eccentric program is that neither immobilization nor rest is necessary, except in very painful cases where athletic activity is impossible. Most athletes with patellar tendinitis have very tight quadriceps (see Fig. 5-7), which may be an etiologic factor.

The basis of the program is to use activities that place maximal stress on the tendon, in order to increase its tensile strength. This is done most readily for the patellar tendon by having the patient drop to a semisquatting position (see Fig. 5-8). The stress on the tendon is increased by adding weight resistance or dropping at a faster rate.

---

5. Jumper's knee

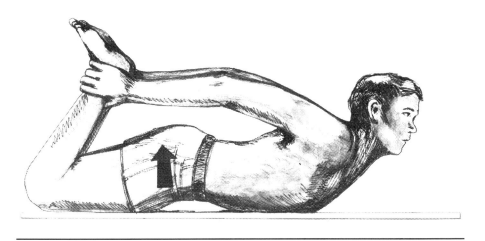

Figure 5-7. Testing for quadriceps tightness: if hip begins to flex as foot is pulled toward buttocks, then these muscles are tight.

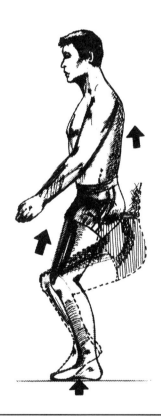

Figure 5-8. Patient drops (or lowers) to a semisquatting position.

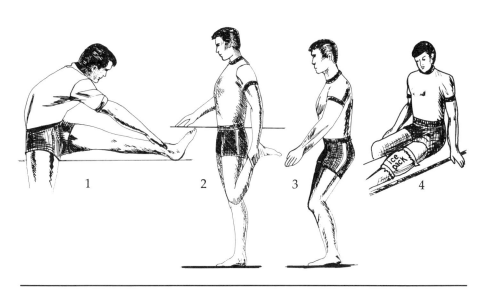

Figure 5-9. The stages of the exercise program: (1) stretch, (2) stretch quads, (3) eccentric exercise, (4) ice (after stretching again).

We are unable to quantitatively assess the loads on the patellar tendon with these variations, but we can use the patient's discomfort as a monitor. The program is outlined in Table 5-5.

"Slow movement" during the eccentric program means a controlled lowering of the body to the semicrouched position and returning it to upright at the same speed. Speed is increased by allowing the body weight to drop more and more rapidly. Finally, patients should be able to allow their body weight to drop freely and stop the movement with eccentric quadriceps contraction. We call this motion *drop and stop*. The patient must understand that the sudden reversal of downward motion is the important feature of the program.

Table 5-5. Eccentric exercise program for jumper's knee
___

1. Warm-up
    a. General, whole-body warm-up
    b. Exercises not involving knee extension
    c. Sufficient when sweating is elicited
2. Stretching
    a. Static stretch of quadriceps and hamstrings
    b. Hold at least 30 seconds
    c. Repeat 3 times
3. Main program
    a. Squatting movements
    b. Focusing primarily on the rapid deceleration phase between the downward and upward movement phase
        Week 1: No added resistance on days 1 and 2 (slow); days 3 to 7 (progressively faster)
        Week 2: Add resistance (10% body weight)
        Weeks 3 to 6: Add 10 to 30 lb progressively
    c. Do three sets of 10 repetitions once daily
    d. After 6 weeks, three sets of 10 three times weekly
4. Warm-down
    a. Static stretch as in item 2
5. Ice
    a. Ice on patellar tendon for 5 minutes after program
6. Optional support
    a. Apply tensor bandage support if desired

___

5. Jumper's knee

As previously explained, no resistance is added until the patient can drop and stop with little or no discomfort. Then the program continues (see Fig. 5-9).

The load on the tendon can be increased further if the athlete drops from a height and the load increases with the drop height. We have not yet had to incorporate this into our program, but this revision may be more feasible than the addition of heavy weights to the shoulders. Also, the movement more closely resembles that used in volleyball and basketball and can be combined with subsequent concentric contraction to practice vertical jumping. Indeed, this method is used by many gymnastics and volleyball coaches to improve jumping ability, especially in Eastern Europe and Russia. They call the technique *depth jumping*, or *plyometrics* (Kovalev 1981; Suwara 1979).

5. Jumper's knee

6. Tennis elbow

Tennis elbow refers to a variety of disorders involving the elbow joint. In fact, more than 25 lesions of this kind have been listed in the literature, including bursitis, arthritis, and neuritis (Priest 1976). The majority of authors, however, seem to agree with Nirschl (1974), who states, "It is our conclusion tht the pathological entity itself is a granulation response to micro-rupture of the extensor carpi radialis brevis and communis aponeurosis at the lateral epicondyle, as well as the subtendinous triangular space at the lateral epicondyle."

We concur with this opinion, but we narrow our definition of tennis elbow to elbow pain that can be related to extensor movements of the wrist joint. These extensors commonly attach to the lateral epicondyle, so the term *lateral epicondylitis* is preferable to *tennis elbow*, especially since the syndrome occurs frequently in nonathletes whose occupations require lots of gripping activities, such as carpenters, fishers, and homemakers.

Structure and function

The lateral epicondyle of the humerus is a point of insertion for the wrist extensors, including extensor carpi radialis longus, extensor carpi radialis brevis, extensor digitorum, and extensor digiti minimi. These muscles attach jointly to the lateral epicondyle via a tendinous expansion known as the common extensor tendon, or extensor aponeurosis (see Fig. 6-1). In addition, the supinator muscle partially attaches to the lateral epicondyle and lies underneath the wrist extensor muscles mentioned above (see Fig. 6-2).

These muscles act to extend the wrist and, in the case of the supinator, to supinate the forearm. The usual activity of the wrist extensors is a synergistic one, whereby the finger flexors contract simultaneously with wrist extension. The positioning of the wrist in extension allows a much more powerful grip. You can easily confirm

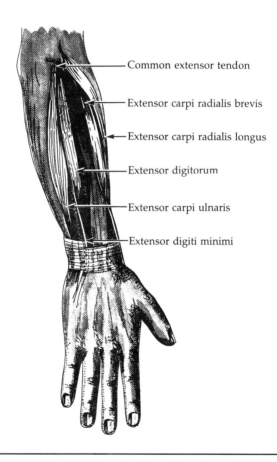

Common extensor tendon

Extensor carpi radialis brevis

Extensor carpi radialis longus

Extensor digitorum

Extensor carpi ulnaris

Extensor digiti minimi

Figure 6-1. The forearm muscles (extensor) that attach to the lateral epicondyle.

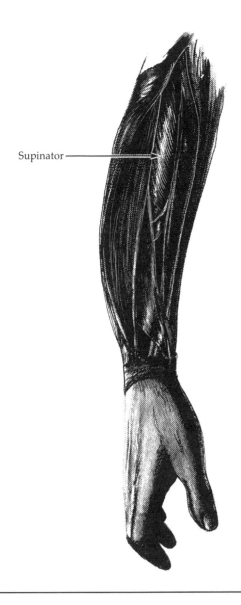

Supinator

Figure 6-2. Supinator lies beneath the wrist extensors, but is intimately connected.

this by attempting to grip an object, first with the wrist extended and then with it flexed. This stabilizing action of the wrist extensors means they are active in virtually all activities requiring use of the hand. The demand increases when stronger gripping is required, whether to hit a backhand at tennis or to use a chain saw.

The ultrastructure of the normal common extensor tendon has not been well studied. However, it can be presumed to be similar to that of other tendinous structures, though it is shorter and thinner than the tendons in the other clinical situations described.

Etiology and mechanics

Despite hundreds of articles throughout the last century, the precise etiology of tennis elbow remains to be clarified. This is the result of the wide range of sources to which the symptoms are attributed. There is agreement, however, that the etiology is probably multifactorial, including one or more of the following:

- Massive overload of extensor muscles
- Multiple repetition of movement
- Quality of tissue
- Age
- Potential hormonal imbalance (in females)
- Strength
- Endurance
- Flexibility
- Mechanics of joint design
- Equipment
- Skill level

We believe that, as in the other cases of chronic tendinitis, the basic etiology of the lesion is the application of forces that exceed the tensile strength of the common extensor tendon. These forces are pro-

6. *Tennis elbow*

duced by the wrist extensors, so any repeated movements involving marked extension movements of the wrist may be responsible. If the tendon is weakened because of previous injury, inflammation, hormonal imbalance, or nutritional deficiency, then it may be more susceptible to damage. Age-related changes may be classified as previous injury, since they are degenerative changes related to repeated microtraumas. This accounts for the high incidence of symptoms in individuals between the ages of 35 and 50 years. In a study of average tennis players, Priest (1976) found that 100 percent of players who had been playing for a number of years were suffering from tennis elbow.

Some authors (Bernhang, Dehner, and Fogarty 1974; Uhthoff and Sarkar 1980) state that poor players or novices are more likely to develop tennis elbow than are more experienced players. They relate this to incorrect technique, particularly on the backhand stroke. Specifically, poor players grip the racket tightly for a longer time than experienced players. They also tend to use their forearm muscles rather than their shoulder muscles and weight transference to hit the ball. This is referred to as the *leading-elbow stroke* (Bernhang, Dehner, and Fogarty 1974) (see Fig. 6-3).

Although this theory seems plausible, there remains the somewhat contradictory evidence that many expert players suffer from tennis elbow as well. Priest et al. (1977) reviewed 84 world-class tennis players and found that 45 percent experienced elbow problems and 37 percent considered their problem severe. In a survey of average players (Priest 1976), 47 percent had elbow pain at some time, and the incidence increased with playing frequency and number of playing years. It seems, therefore, that different factors contribute to tennis elbow. Poor stroke mechanics and muscle weakness are at fault in the beginner, while factors such as excessive string tension, fatigue owing to repeated loading, inflexibility, and occasional mishits cause the disorder in experienced players.

---

6. Tennis elbow

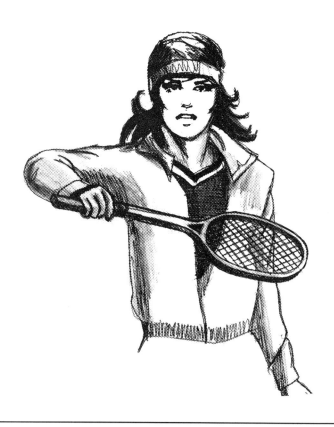

Figure 6-3. The leading-elbow stroke.

Bernhang, Dehner, and Fogarty (1974) measured the grip force, racquet bending strain, and EMG activity of the wrist extensors during tennis strokes. They found increased activity in the extensors during the anticipatory phase of the backhand stroke and an impact stretching of the muscles as the ball hit the racquet. These actions produced a stretch reflex in the muscle and an eccentric contraction. Hitting the ball off center markedly increases the extensor activity and creates torque at the elbow. The combination of impact stretch and torque appears particularly likely to cause injury. The phenomenon of stretch seems important in the etiology, since symptoms are more likely to occur if the forearm is pronated, a position that stretches the wrist extensors. You can easily see the reduced flexibility of the wrist extensors of the dominant side if you attempt to flex both wrists while holding forearms extended and pronated.

The mention of torque brings us to another point frequently debated in the discussion of tennis elbow, that of optimum grip size. Bernhang, Dehner, and Fogarty (1974) attempted to control torque with different grip sizes and found that torque control improved with increasing grip size. They concluded that the grip size should be as large as is comfortably possible.

Another sport particularly likely to cause tennis elbow is squash. The racquet grip is much smaller, and wrist extensor action is required more constantly since the wrist should be cocked throughout both forehand and backhand strokes. Players with a "wristy backhand" or who are playing a lob from the front of the court are especially vulnerable. Nonetheless, fewer squash players are afflicted, probably because of the lighter racquets used. Badminton players fall in the same category as squash players. They use even more wrist extension, but the racquet is very light so they are less susceptible to lateral epicondylitis (see Fig. 6-4).

---

6. Tennis elbow

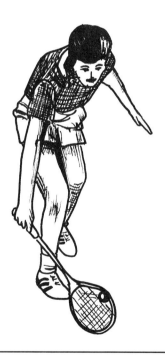

Figure 6-4. A backhand stroke near the front of the squash court.

The same principles just described for tennis players apply to others as well. Repeated loading over an extended period or a sudden increase in use of the wrist extensors (such as in renovating a house) may cause tennis elbow in nonathletes.

Signs and symptoms

The symptoms of lateral epicondylitis are pain on strong gripping action and weakness of the grip as a result of pain. The signs are tenderness with pressure on the point of the lateral epicondyle, pain and weakness with resisted wrist extension, and pain on stretching of the wrist extensors (see Fig. 6-5).

Pathology

The use of surgery as a treatment for resistant cases of lateral epicondylitis offers a means by which the pathologic changes occurring in the common extensor tendon may be examined. Such reports are numerous in the literature (Cyriax 1936; Boyd and McLeod 1973; Nirschl 1974; Nirschl and Pettrone 1979; Uhthoff and Sarkar 1980). Specimens of excised tissue show scattered areas of thinning and fibrillation of fiber bundles, with microruptures of tendinous bundles. These microruptures were not discernible during surgery, but are characterized by a break in the axial arrangement of the fibers with the break filled by amorphous debris. They are accompanied by fibroblastic cell reaction and vascular proliferation. You will recognize this as the response to tendon injury outlined in Chapter 2: tendon overuse results in microscopic rupture and subsequent tendinous nonrepair with immature tissue.

6. *Tennis elbow*

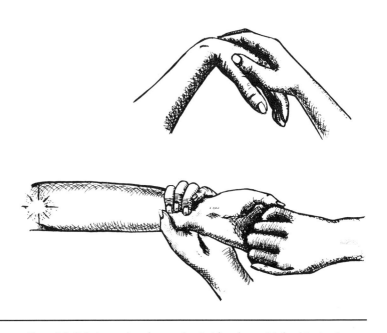

Figure 6-5. Pain is experienced on passive stretch and on resisted wrist extension.

The number of structures described by various authors as being the underlying pathology in tennis elbow is extensive. Cyriax compiled a list in 1936 which is just as diverse today and included the following:

1. Traumatic periostitis
2. Arthritis, synovitis, sprain, adhesions, or torn capsule of the radiohumeral joint
3. Arthritis, synovitis, sprain, or adhesions of the radioulnar joint
4. Displaced, frayed, torn, or inflamed orbicular ligament
5. Sprained, torn radial collateral ligament
6. Inflamed radiohumeral bursa
7. Inflamed subcutaneous epicondylar bursa
8. Nipped synovial fringe in radiohumeral or radioulnar joint
9. Tear or fibrositis of extensor origin
10. Tear or fibrositis of supinator
11. Torn pronator teres
12. Torn extensor carpi radialis longus
13. Torn extensor carpi radialis brevis
14. Tear of brachioradialis
15. Tear of extensor digitorum communis
16. Myositis or tear of extensor muscles
17. Torn anconeus
18. Radial incongruence
19. Rheumatism, gout, influenzal sequelae, focal sepsis
20. Neuritis of radial, posterior interosseous, or antebrachial cutaneous nerves
21. Osteochondritis

Priest (1976) mentions that more than 43 separate pathologies may be found in the literature. You may well be daunted by the prospect of having to distinguish between so many possible causes of pain. However, evidence points to tears of the common extensor tendon as being by far the most common reason for symptoms. Since we also felt this is true, we assume this diagnosis if the physical signs are appropriate and pursue treatment accordingly. Should the patient fail to respond, further investigation can prove necessary.

6. Tennis elbow

Structures in and around the elbow may be involved secondary to the original lesion, so the underlying cause may not appear to be the primary one.

Treatment

In view of the diversity of opinion regarding the etiology of tennis elbow, it is not surprising to find an equally vast array of treatment techniques. The list includes rest, cast immobilization, steroid injection, systemic anti-inflammatories, ice, ultrasound, heat, deep friction, manipulation, bracing, and surgery. Although any of these methods may prove successful under certain circumstances, the very existence of such variety and the number of patients who have experienced many of, or all, these treatment techniques should serve as convincing evidence that none is entirely successful.

In his examination of expert tennis players, Priest (1976) could reach no conclusion regarding the efficacy of treatment the players had experienced because of the number of types each had undergone.

In his attempt to consolidate the various treatments, Nirschl (1974) presented a good review of treatment concepts:

1. Relief of acute inflammation
2. Relief of chronic inflammation
3. Increasing forearm muscle power, flexibility, and endurance
4. Decreasing the moment of force at the elbow:
   a. Alter sport
   b. Change equipment
   c. Use an elbow support
5. Surgery if conservative treatment fails

Our treatment does not differ greatly from this regime. We advocate the liberal use of ice and sometimes oral anti-inflammatory drugs to control inflammation. Brief periods of rest may be necessary in acute cases. The use of a forearm brace (see Fig. 6-6) is also suggested to relieve symptoms during the treatment period. The exact mecha-

6. Tennis elbow

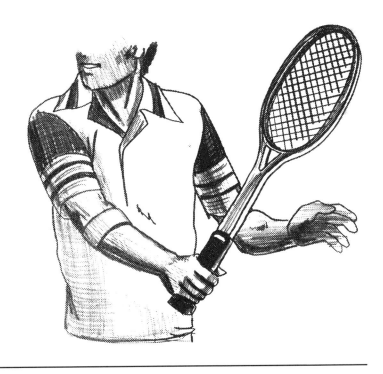

Figure 6-6. Use of a forearm band to relieve symptoms.

nism of action of this brace is unclear, but it appears to function by providing a reactive counterforce against the contracting muscles and either spreads the force over a wider area or decreases the contractile pull on the lateral epicondyle. The brace is applied snugly to the relaxed forearm just prior to activity and is removed immediately afterward.

The main difference in our approach to the treatment of tennis elbow lies in our emphasis on exercise. This stems from the knowledge that decreased flexibility causes the muscles to be overstretched during eccentric contraction and overloading of the extensors is the most widely recognized factor in the etiology of the syndrome. Maximum strengthening of the muscle must necessarily include eccentric exercise, since this is the nature of the force producing the injury and since eccentric exercise produces greater tensile force on the tendon.

Control of loading on the muscle is carried out in the same manner as previously described, that is, by altering the speed of movement or the amount of resistance. We suggest a starting weight of 2 lb (1 lb for females) in acute cases and 5 lb in less severe cases. Warm-up may be effectively provided by local heat application for a few minutes or by general body exercise.

The patient stretches the wrist extensors by pronating the forearm with the elbow extended and then passively flexing the wrist. This flexing may be done with the opposite hand or by placing the flexed hand on a support of a suitable level (see Fig. 6-7).

Following three 30-second stretches, the patient sits with the forearm supported so that the hand and weight are beyond the support. Then the weight may be lowered and raised freely. Again, the emphasis is on the change from downward to upward motion. The exercise is repeated 30 times, in three sets of 10 (see Fig. 6-8). The stretching exercises are repeated, and ice is applied to the lateral epicondyle. One very convenient method of doing this is to freeze a

6. Tennis elbow

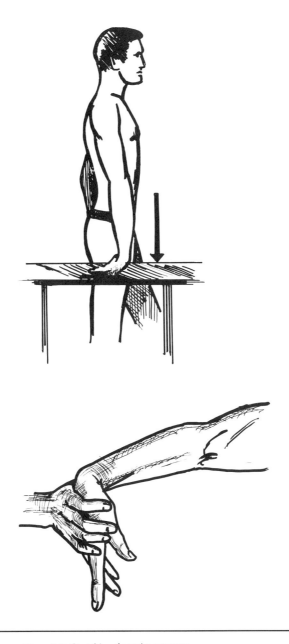

Figure 6-7. Stretching the wrist extensors.

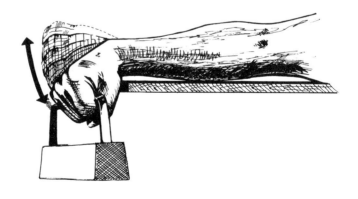

Figure 6-8. With forearm supported, lower weight over the side.

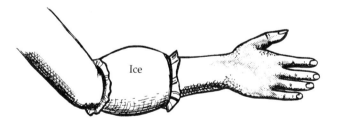

Figure 6-9. Final stage: apply ice.

paper cup full of water and use this to rub gently over the area for 5 minutes. It may be placed back in the freezer and reused. Alternatively, an ice cube with a stick frozen inside it or crushed ice in a damp towel may be used (see Fig. 6-9).

The entire session should take about 20 minutes and is done daily. As with Achilles and patellar tendinitides, it may be 2 or 3 weeks before symptoms begin to abate. During this interval the patient should be checked regularly to ensure the program is done regularly and correctly and progresses when indicated. The yardstick of discomfort (or absence of same) near the end of 30 repetitions determines when the speed or resistance should be changed.

6. Tennis elbow

7. *Other tendinitides*

In the previous three chapters we discussed the most commonly seen types of tendinitis: Achilles tendinitis, patellar tendinitis, and lateral epicondylitis. We also explained the reasoning behind our theory that eccentric muscle contraction is the most important etiologic factor in these cases. Yet, as the clinician knows all too well, there are numerous other tendinitides that can be equally difficult to treat. The purpose of this chapter is to review some of these disorders, their etiologies, and possible avenues of treatment. We should emphasize that we do *not* advocate the use of eccentric exercise in treating all types of tendinitis. Similarly, you should not assume that all the clinical entities mentioned in this chapter are necessarily amenable to treatment with eccentric exercise. Where this is true, we indicate it. Otherwise, we present what we feel is the best method of treatment or the most widely used.

Upper limb

Shoulder and shoulder girdle

SUPRASPINATUS TENDINITIS   This is the most common type of tendinitis in the upper limb. It occurs most frequently in swimmers and tennis players or athletes in any other sport requiring repeated overhead movement of the arm.

Knowledge of the anatomy of the shoulder joint and supraspinatus tendon is essential for understanding this injury. The supraspinatus tendon passes beneath the acromion and inserts on the greater tubercle of the humerus, passing beneath the coracoacromial ligament which forms a fibrous arch over the tendon. Between the tendon and the overlying structures is the subacromial bursa.

Repeated abduction of the shoulder, unless it is maintained in external rotation, causes impingement of the tendon within the very narrow space between the humerus and the overlying acromion and ligament. This disorder is often referred to as *impingement syndrome.* You can readily see how the free-style stroke in swimming can cause this disorder, which has a second nickname, *swimmer's shoulder.*

Rathbun and MacNab (1970) studied the microvasculature of the supraspinatus tendon and found it to be reduced where the tendon was "wrung out" by pressure during abduction (see Fig. 7-1). This site corresponds to that of tears in the supraspinatus of older patients. Therefore, the authors postulated that these tears were the result of poor healing owing to impaired circulation. Although tears are not as common in younger patients, the area affected is the same. Sometimes calcification occurs at the site.

The etiology of this type of tendinitis is well defined and can be confirmed by horizontally adducting the patient's arm across the body. This move causes further impingement and reproduces the painful symptoms.

Eccentric exercise is *not* indicated in this type of tendinitis. The methods we employ include ice, stretching exercises, gradual warm-up, change of stroke and/or reduction in practice distance, anti-inflammatory drugs, and (in some cases) surgical release of the overlying coracoacromial ligament.

BICIPITAL TENDINITIS   The long head of the biceps arises by a long, narrow tendon from the supraglenoid tubercle of the scapula. The long head passes through the shoulder joint and emerges from it to lie in the intertubercular sulcus (bicipital groove) where it is restrained by the transverse humeral ligament (see Fig. 7-2). Thus, it is subject to the same type of impingement as the supraspinatus tendon; indeed, it may be difficult at first to differentiate between the two. One distinguishing feature relates to internal and external rotation of the shoulder. During abduction, rotation is usually painful

7. Other tendinitides

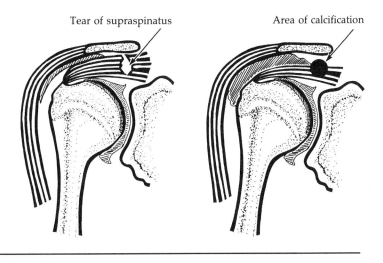

Figure 7-1. Sites of supraspinatus tendinitis.

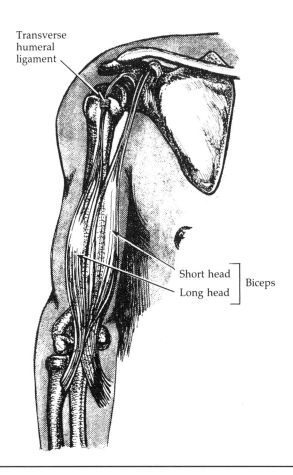

Transverse
humeral
ligament

Short head ⎤
Long head ⎦ Biceps

Figure 7-2. Anatomy of the bicipital tendon.

in cases of bicipital tendinitis, especially if the examiner applies slight pressure with the fingers to the tendon in its groove while the arm is passively maneuvered. In patients with supraspinatus tendinitis, the internally rotated position may be painful, but this pain will disappear when the humerus is rotated outward because the greater tubercle of the humerus no longer impinges on the acromion process.

The slight differences in the mechanics of these two types of tendinitis mean that bicipital tendinitis occurs more often in athletes who participate in sports involving throwing or paddling. Of course, bicipital tendinitis may occur in swimmers and other athletes as well, sometimes secondary to supraspinatus tendinitis since the ensuing inflammation may involve the nearby biceps.

Treatment is usually aimed at relieving the inflammation and pressure on the tendon by means of ice, anti-inflammatory drugs, or a steroid injection into the tendon sheath. These conservative methods are nearly always successful.

TRICEPS TENDINITIS   The attachment of the long head of the triceps to the infraglenoid tubercle of the scapula, where it blends into the capsule of the shoulder joint, is sometimes a site of triceps tendinitis. Pain is produced by vigorous throwing and can be reproduced during examination by extending the shoulder with the elbow flexed and having the patient attempt to extend the elbow against resistance (see Fig. 7-3).

7. Other tendinitides

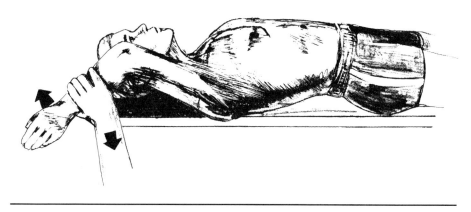

Figure 7-3. Stretching the triceps muscles (elbow must be flexed and shoulder extended as far as possible).

The depth of this lesion and the covering of other muscles make it difficult to treat with ice, physiotherapy, or injection. Indeed, it proves very resistant to treatment and often recurs. We recommend strengthening the muscle eccentrically by having the patient exercise as shown in Figure 7-4. The difficulty in performing these exercises adequately alone may make supervision and assistance from a therapist necessary.

Other shoulder girdle muscles

The infraspinatus and teres minor may be injured during racquet sports that require rotation of the shoulder, for example, squash. Treatment with stretching and resisted exercises, plus physiotherapeutic modalities to relieve symptoms, works rapidly in these cases.

Less commonly, the scapular attachment of the teres major becomes painful, usually as a result of throwing. The symptoms are similar to those in triceps tendinitis, except that pain is reproduced by having the patient lie supine, with the arm abducted and fully externally rotated, and internally rotate the arm against manual resistance.

In general, any muscle-tendon unit may give rise to pain, depending on the sport and the individual characteristics of the athlete. If doubt exists as to the muscle involved, careful positioning so that each muscle is placed in a lengthened position and made to contract against resistance can be helpful in identifying the specific muscle. The positions can be found in manuals of muscle testing (e.g., Daniels and Worthingham 1972).

Elbow

The most common disorder here is, of course, tennis elbow (discussed in Chapter 6). Less common is tendinitis of the common flexor tendon, for which the phrase *golfer's elbow* has been coined. The etiology is much the same as that of tennis elbow, and treatment is similar except that the direction of motion is reversed.

7. Other tendinitides

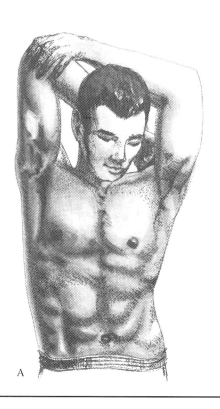

A

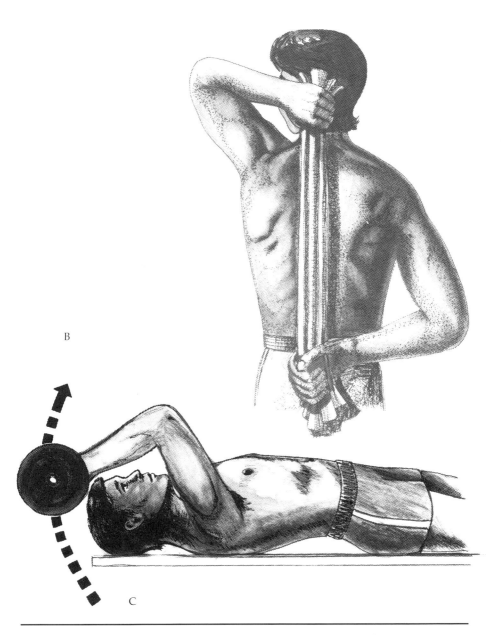

B

C

Figure 7-4. A,B. *Two methods of stretching the triceps.* C. *The eccentric exercise program.*

Wrist	Excessive, repetitive movements of, or pressure on, the wrist extensor tendons may inflame the tendon sheaths as they pass under the extensor retinaculum (see Fig. 7-5). Most commonly affected are the tendons of the abductor pollicis longus and extensor pollicis brevis, which occupy the same synovial sheath and pass in a bony groove behind the radiostyloid process to form a sharp angle and insert on the thumb. Synovitis results from friction between the tendon and its sheath and the bony process and the overlying retinaculum. The symptoms are aching discomfort over the styloid process, aggravated by movements of the wrist and thumb, and pain on stretching the tendons or resisted thumb abduction. Treatment usually consists of local ice application, anti-inflammatory drugs, and physiotherapy (usually ultrasound in water). These measures are nearly always successful, although sometimes steroid injections or (more rarely) surgery may be necessary in very resistant cases.

Lower limb	The muscle-tendon units of the lower limb are subjected to greater force than those of the upper limb because of the larger masses (limb or body) that they must move. Also more regular activity is required of these muscles both in daily activity (e.g., walking) and in sports. The most common tendinitides of the lower limb, Achilles tendinitis and jumper's knee, have been discussed (in Chapters 4 and 5, respectively). Here we present some other lower limb lesions that can occur, focusing on those in which eccentric contraction contributes to the etiology.

Groin injury

Groin injuries include lesions in a number of muscles of the upper thigh, namely iliopsoas, rectus femoris, sartorius, pectineus, adductor brevis, gracilis, and so on. These muscles are illustrated in Figure 7-6. The action of these muscles (hip flexion and adduction) means they are used commonly in kicking. They are also stretched when the hip joint is abducted and/or extended. Injury to these muscles

7. Other tendinitides

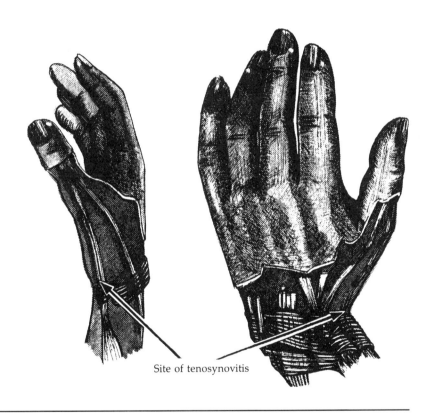

Site of tenosynovitis

Figure 7-5. De Quervain's syndrome due to increased pressure.

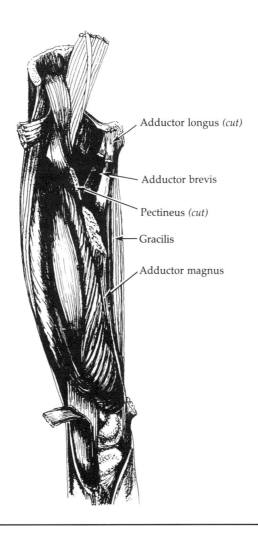

Adductor longus *(cut)*

Adductor brevis

Pectineus *(cut)*

Gracilis

Adductor magnus

Figure 7-6. Adductor muscles.

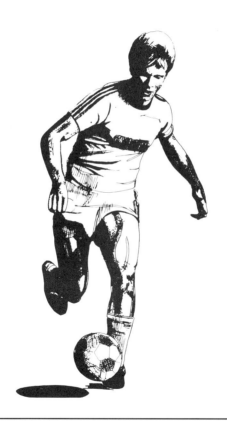

Figure 7-7. Leg changes from backward to forward, causing stretch in hip flexors and adductors.

occurs most frequently in soccer players, a not unusual finding in light of the action of these muscles and the use of the lower limbs in this sport.

In kicking, first the hip is extended. Then this motion is arrested, and the hip is suddenly flexed (see Fig. 7-7). At this point the iliopsoas and rectus femoris are contracting eccentrically. Also the adductor muscles of the opposite limb must contract to maintain the horizontal position of the pelvis, especially if the player stops suddenly while running or changes direction. The fixing of the foot to the ground that occurs with the wearing of cleats may contribute to the stretching of the adductor muscles. The second sport in which groin injuries commonly occur is ice hockey. The sliding of a skate laterally on the ice easily causes the adductor muscles to be overstretched.

The symptoms of a *groin pull,* as these injuries are usually called, are pain on movements requiring stretch and/or contraction of the muscle (such as kicking or changing direction during skating or running). The pain may be severe enough to prevent the player from participating in sports. You can test clinically for this disorder by placing the hip in an abducted and slightly extended position and having the patient attempt to both flex and adduct the thigh simultaneously. It is important to have the patient initiate both muscle actions, since these movements performed singly often will *not* cause symptoms (see Fig. 7-8).

The combined flexion and adduction movement, with resistance added, is used in treatment. Since it is difficult to apply external weight resistance (although ankle weights may be used), frequently the assistance of another person is required. Usually this is the therapist, since the exercise will be quite painful if it is done improperly and supervision is required. The treatment program follows a common pattern: warm-up, stretch, resisted exercises, stretch, and ice application. Because of the difficulty (and discomfort) in applying ice in some cases, it may be omitted if desired.

---

7. Other tendinitides

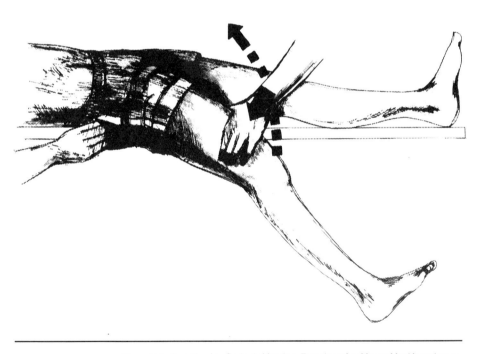

Figure 7-8. Resisting hip flexion/adduction. Examiner should stand beside patient to get best angle and to give security against falling.

Muscle tightness appears to be especially at fault in these injuries, since soccer and hockey players are, in our experience, notoriously inflexible. Hip flexors should be tested for tightness (see Fig. 7-9), and special emphasis laid on flexibility exercises during treatment.

In order to have a definitive diagnosis of the groin injury, it is important to remember to isolate muscles one at a time. Position them so they are stretched; then resist their contraction in the lengthened position. Usually the affected muscle-tendon unit can be easily identified in this manner. Table 7-1 provides some common positions for testing various muscles of the thigh. Most physiotherapists are very adept at selective muscle testing and should be consulted if any uncertainty remains.

Hamstrings pull

The hamstrings, namely the biceps femoris, semitendinosus, and semimembranosus (see Fig. 7-10), originate on the ischial tuberosity and insert on the tibia and fibula. They flex the knee, can act in hip extension, and are stretched by flexing the hip with the knee straight. During lower limb motion, the hamstrings contract eccentrically to decelerate the leg in the last part of the swing-through phase of gait. This activity increases as the speed of the leg increases, as in running and kicking. Indeed, it is during explosive running activities that the hamstrings are most often injured. Hurdlers would appear to be particularly vulnerable because of the extreme stretch put on the hamstrings (see Fig. 7-11); however, sprinters are injured most often. There are probably two reasons for this: (1) higher tensions in the hamstrings during the decelerative phase of lower leg motion in the forward recovery of the swinging limb and (2) less attention to flexibility.

Treatment of hamstring injuries is aimed at strengthening and stretching the muscle. The strengthening is done as the patient lies prone and lowers a weight from knee flexion to extension, then *immediately* flexes again. This may be done on a Universal gym.

---

7. Other tendinitides

Table 7-1. Common positions for testing thigh muscles

Muscle	Action	Position of patient	Test
Rectus femoris	Flex hip and extend knee	Supine	Flex hip with knee straight
Iliopsoas	Flex hip	Supine at edge of bed so hip can extend in neutral plane	Flex hip, allowing knee flexion
Sartorius	Flex hip and knee, externally rotate hip	Sitting over edge of plinth	Have patient flex hip while bringing knee to shoulder on same side
Pectineus, adductor brevis[a]	Adduct hip	Supine with leg slightly extended	Resist adduction in horizontal plane
Adductor longus, magnus	Adduct hip	Supine with leg abducted and knee flexed	Resist adduction in horizontal plane
Gracilis	Adduct hip, flex knee, medially rotate thigh	Supine with leg abducted and knee straight	Attempt to laterally rotate thigh while person resists (applying resistance at heel will bring knee flexion)

[a]Since pectineus and adductor brevis are shorter muscles, less hip abduction is necessary to stretch them. Also, pectineus and adductor brevis originate more anteriorly on the pubis and so may be stretched farther by placing the hip in extension.

7. Other tendinitides

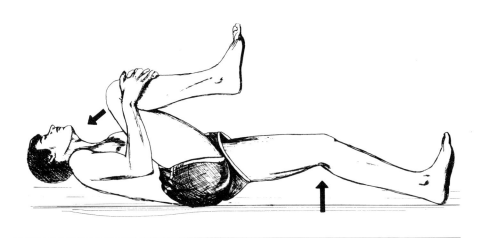

Figure 7-9. Testing for hip flexor tightness. Flex one knee to the chest. If the other leg lifts from the bed, the hip flexors are tight.

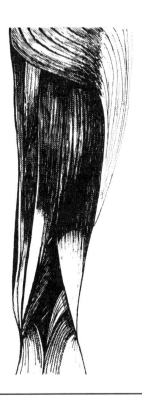

Figure 7-10. Hamstring muscles of the back of the thigh.

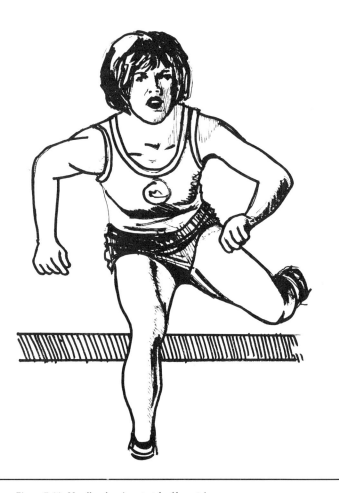

Figure 7-11. Hurdler showing stretch of hamstrings.

Assistance may be necessary to prevent the knee from "snapping" into extension when heavy weights are being used, or a small cushion or rolled towel may be placed beneath the ankle as it strikes the table to relieve any apprehension on the patient's part. Proprioceptive neuromuscular facilitation (PNF) techniques, combining stretching and contracting (see Fig. 7-12), are particularly effective for these injuries but require a partner. As with groin injuries, special emphasis should be placed on flexibility in treatment for hamstring injuries.

Shin splints

Shin splints is another term that actually encompasses a number of different clinical entities, including posterior tibial tendinitis, anterior tibial tendinitis, anterior compartment syndrome, deep posterior compartment syndrome, and tendinitis of other deep calf muscles. The symptoms are pain in the middle one-third of the leg and tenderness along the interosseous border of the tibia.

This injury occurs most commonly in runners who are not using properly cushioned shoes or who run on hard surfaces. It is frequently seen in tennis and basketball players also. In long-distance runners, shin splints are associated with excessive forefoot pronation, that is, flat feet. This flattening of the medial longitudinal arch stretches the tibialis posterior muscle which inverts the foot and elevates the medial longitudinal arch.

Treatment for shin splints consists of reducing training mileage, anti-inflammatory drugs, local ice application, and construction of an orthotic to maintain the position of the medial longitudinal arch. Orthotics need not be complicated and may be purchased at the local drug store. (Advice against this indicates a more complex problem.)

When tightness of the muscles is suspected, having the patient stand on one foot and bend at the knee stretches the deep posterior

7. Other tendinitides

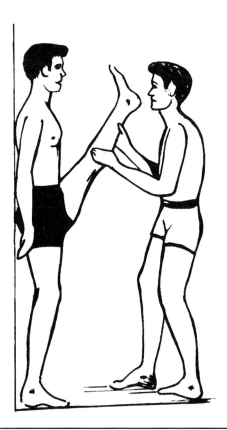

Figure 7-12. Stretching the hamstrings. Take leg upward until limit is reached, then have patient try to push leg down toward bed while you resist. Then patient relaxes, and you push the limb farther.

muscles. These are the muscles that, if tight, prevent dorsiflexion of the ankle. This stretching exercise should be part of any stretching routine; it is illustrated in Figure 4-5 (p. 87). The bent knee emphasizes stretching of the soleus, posterior tibial, and flexor muscles.

Tendinitis of the anterior tibial muscles is frequently referred to as shin splints but is easily differentiated because of the different location of pain. In true shin splints, pain occurs in the middle third of the leg; the pain in tendinitis of the anterior tibial muscles occurs in the upper third of the anterolateral aspect of the leg.

Compartment syndrome

The leg is divided into three compartments: the *anterior,* containing the tibialis anterior, extensor digitorum longus, peroneus longus, extensor hallucis longus, and peroneus brevis muscles; the *deep posterior,* containing the flexor hallucis longus, flexor digitorum longus, and tibialis posterior muscles; and the *superficial posterior,* containing gastrocnemius and soleus muscles. Injury to a compartment causes swelling, which can occlude the blood supply to the nerves and muscle contained within it. Since each compartment is bounded by a tight fascial sheath, the swelling leads to a rise in pressure within the compartment and subsequent occlusion. This is *compartment syndrome.* Enlargement of the muscle without previous injury also can lead to symptoms. This usually occurs in the anterior compartment and causes impairment of function of the anterolateral muscles of the leg and of the deep peroneal nerve. The symptoms are weakness of toe extension and ankle dorsiflexion and numbness in the cleft between the first and second toes. Compartment syndrome most often occurs in runners. It often disappears spontaneously after some time, but a favorite surgical treatment is to divide the overlying fascia (fasciotomy), thereby relieving the pressure. The results of surgery, however, are equivocal. Symptoms recur in many cases, and up to a 15 percent loss in strength may occur (Garfin et al. 1981). Nonetheless, fasciotomy in cases of compartment syndrome following lower limb trauma is considered an emergency.

7. Other tendinitides

Conclusion Therapists and physicians frequently encounter numerous other disorders occurring in the lower limb during sports participation that we have not discussed in other chapters in this book. In most instances, these disorders are related to trauma and so are outside the scope of this book. The cases that fall outside this classification are presented in this chapter for purposes of differential diagnosis only. Where eccentric exercise is involved, we have outlined the exercise program that should be used.

Again, we would like to emphasize careful history taking, since this will tell the examiner both the injured structure and the reason for injury. Selective examination to determine the exact site of injury may be necessary and is important in isolating the muscle group at fault and exercising it correctly. In areas where several muscles perform similar functions, a noninjured muscle will perform the task unless the injured muscle-tendon unit is isolated.

Although we feel that eccentric contraction is involved in many cases of lower limb muscle injuries, particularly hamstring and groin pulls, there are equal numbers where eccentric activity is not involved. We advise you to be discriminating in applying this treatment.

8. *Clinical results*

The development of the eccentric exercise program was prompted by our disappointment with traditional treatment methods and the growing realization that we were not employing our knowledge of the behavior of soft tissue under different physical conditions. Dr. Howard Lamb, research fellow at the Nova Scotia Sport Medicine Clinic in 1978, questioned our "standard" treatment of tendinitis, which at that time consisted of physical modalities, oral anti-inflammatories, flexibility exercises, ice application, transcutaneous neurologic stimulation (TNS), and so forth. Dr. Lamb reasoned that the tensile strength of the tendon was being exceeded during activity and that this action was causing the microruptures that led to injury. Moreover, he felt that only by addressing the problem of tensile strength instability directly would it be solved. That is, the tendon must be gradually and progressively overloaded, thereby increasing its tensile strength. Immobility or disuse of the tendon (and, in fact, all soft tissues) simply weakened it. Thus, we encouraged our patients to remain active, and we avoided the use of rest as a treatment modality except where absolutely necessary.

Yet we failed to take measures to strengthen the tendon. The stretching and isometric and concentric exercises that we prescribed did not produce enough tensile force on the tendon. Dr. Lamb pointed this out and said we should be using eccentric loading for two reasons:

1. It simulated actual movements involved in the sport.
2. It produced more tensile force than other forms of exercise.

Thus our eccentric exercise program was born. To examine the efficacy of the program, we surveyed 200 patients who had been thus treated. Although patients with varying types of tendinitis had been seen, we decided to review those with Achilles tendinitis, patellar tendinitis, or lateral epicondylitis because they made up the largest percentage of our patient population. The histories were documented and the diagnoses confirmed by three separate observers: the orthopedist, the research fellow, and the physiotherapist. Each patient was given specific instruction in how to perform the exercises and was checked regularly by the therapist to ensure that they were done correctly and that the patient progressed appropriately.

After initial instruction, each patient was issued an instruction manual and a diary for recording daily exercise. The program was modified according to each patient's problem and the severity of symptoms at initial evaluation. We have emphasized the importance of selecting the appropriate speed of movement and amount of resistance, and this was carefully explained to each patient. Each patient's manual contained an illustrated and written description of the specific program to be carried out.

Patient
description

The group of 200 patients contained 136 males and 64 females, distributed across the three categories of injuries. Their age groups are shown in Table 8-1. The age distribution is fairly even, except for a greater number of individuals in the category of 36 to 40 years. This is in accordance with the higher incidence of tendinitis said to occur

Table 8-1. Age distribution of tendinitis patients
treated with eccentric exercise program

Age group (yrs)	Number of patients
10–15	6
16–20	35
21–25	31
26–30	28
31–35	27
36–40	56
41–50	17

8. Clinical results

in the fourth decade of life. The importance of degeneration owing to aging as a likely precursor to chronic tendinitis, suggested by a number of researchers, was not apparent in our study population. The group of patients 41 to 50 years old had fewer, not more, individuals.

Symptoms

The patients were examined and diagnosed on their initial visit to the Nova Scotia Sport Medicine Clinic. At that time, a history of their current and past symptoms was obtained. The mean duration of symptoms, and secondary functional limitation, was 18 months, with a range from 6 months to 10 years. Thus, all patients clearly fell within the category defined as chronic tendinitis.

The severity of symptoms as perceived by the individual prior to the program was recorded according to this classification:

Mild	Pain with activity, not interfering with athletic performance
Moderate	Pain of sufficient magnitude to hinder sports activity and decrease performance
Severe	Pain preventing athletic performance. The number of patients in each group, both before and after treatment, is presented in Table 8-2.

Sports activity

All our patients were actively involved in athletics prior to beginning the program, except when their pain had reached a level that prevented them from participating. Even in these cases, patients were frequently involved in some activity other than that which produced their symptoms. For example, a runner with Achilles tendinitis may have switched to swimming or bicycling, or a tennis player with lateral epicondylitis may have been limited to running. We encouraged all patients to participate in sports, allowing the level of discomfort to dictate the level of this participation. Thus, the treatment program did not alter the patient's regular lifestyle. The amount of athletic

8. Clinical results

activity was estimated by each patient (see Table 8-3). The majority were involved quite vigorously in athletics, 80 percent for more than 1 hour daily.

We examined each patient group to determine which sports were responsible for provoking symptoms. The results are presented in Table 8-4. These data support the views that Achilles tendinitis is associated with running, patellar tendinitis with jumping sports, and lateral epicondylitis with tennis. Thus, the eponyms *jumper's knee* and *tennis elbow* are, indeed, very appropriate.

Table 8-2. Severity of symptoms in tendinitis patients
before and after eccentric exercise program

Level	Description	Number of patients		Percentage of patients	
		Before	After	Before	After
Mild	Pain with activity, not hampering athletic activity	30	96	15	48
Moderate	Pain of sufficient magnitude to hinder performance	111	10	56	5
Severe	Pain preventing athletic performance	59	4	29	2
Pain-free		0	90	0	45

8. Clinical results

Table 8-3. Hours of athletic activity per week in
tendinitis patients on eccentric exercise program

Hours	Number of patients	Percentage of patients
<5	40	20
6–10	110	55
>10	50	25

Table 8-4. Sports responsible for tendon disorder

Achilles tendinitis
   Running, 40%
   Jumping, 35%
   Racquet sports, 20%
   Other, 5%
Patellar tendinitis
   Volleyball and basketball, 75%
   Gymnastics, 15%
   Figure skating, 5%
   Other, 5%
Tennis elbow
   Tennis, 60%
   Racquetball, 20%
   Other (rare in squash), 20%

8. Clinical results

Because of the length of duration of symptoms, we expected to find that many patients had undergone previous treatment. We discovered that all patients had received some other form of treatment, often more than one. On average, each patient had undergone six separate programs of treatment, with an average duration of 2 weeks per treatment. This confirmed the lack of success with traditional conservative treatment methods that we and others had experienced.

The program sequence is as outlined in previous chapters. It is designed to be done once daily (minimum) for 6 weeks. Of our patients, 20 percent felt it was necessary to do the exercises twice daily.

The mean follow-up time was 16 months, so that many patients had completed the program by the time of the survey. We were able to determine the time each patient spent on the program by examining the diaries and by patient response to the survey (see Table 8-5).

To determine how effective the program was, we asked patients to rate their response to the program in the following way:

Excellent	Complete relief of symptoms (44%)
Good	Marked decrease in pain and functional disability (43.5%)
Poor	No change in symptoms (9.5%)
Very poor	Symptoms made worse (2%)

Thus, nearly 90 percent of patients had good or excellent results, even though only 30 percent stayed on the program the entire 6 weeks. Many patients stopped the program before 6 weeks because their symptoms either disappeared or diminished to the point where they no longer interfered with activity. When questioned concerning their pain during sports, 45 percent of patients were completely normal, 48 percent were experiencing minimal pain

8. Clinical results

without altered performance, and 7 percent were still hampered during athletics. The results of the program for each type of tendinitis are presented in Table 8-6.

Note that those suffering from patellar tendinitis seemed to respond least well to the program, in that only 30 percent experienced complete relief of symptoms and four patients felt their symptoms were made worse. However, because of the varying lengths of follow-up, some patients were still pursuing the program and may have not reached the point where a reduction in symptoms might be expected. Since patients maintain full activity, an increase in symptoms during the first 2 to 3 weeks of the program is not unusual.

Table 8-5. Time tendinitis patients spent on eccentric exercise program

Time	Percentage of patients
Less than 5 weeks	65
6–8 weeks	30
More than 8 weeks	5

Table 8-6. Improvement in symptoms experienced by tendinitis patients on eccentric exercise program

	Patellar tendinitis		Achilles tendinitis		Tennis elbow (lateral epicondylitis)	
	Number	Percentage	Number	Percentage	Number	Percentage
Complete relief	20	30.3	31	54.4	39	50.6
Marked decrease in symptoms	42	63.6	26	45.6	19	24.7
No change	0	0	0	0	19	24.7
Symptoms worse	4	6.1	0	0	0	0

8. Clinical results

Discussion   The results of this study are not intended to be viewed as those of a controlled clinical trial comparing eccentric exercise with other modalities, but rather as descriptive data to assess the general efficacy of eccentric exercise plus continuing physical activity in the treatment of chronic tendinitis. Since all patients had undergone previous different forms of treatment, they would not have been suitable for a controlled trial. Our results are presented here so that the reader can see why we have been encouraged to use this program routinely in the treatment of chronic tendinitis.

The advantages of the eccentric program are several. Chief among them is the fact that patients are not required to cease athletic activity during the treatment period. The psychological and physiologic effects of interrupting a training program are well known. For the athlete in midseason, this interruption can be viewed as disastrous and often results in poor patient compliance. Other advantages include the following:

1. *Training effect.* Both muscle and tendon are increased in strength as a result of overloading.
2. *Flexibility.* The "tightness" of many athletes is probably a causative factor in these, and other, injuries. The incorporation of stretching in the program promotes increased flexibility.
3. *Ease of performance.* The program is short and takes only about 20 to 30 minutes to perform. We suggest it be done at a time some hours from or (if this is not possible) prior to practice since the discomfort from physical activity may result in the incorrect amount of resistance being applied.
4. *No supervision necessary.* The ability of patients to carry out the program independently saves time for both patient and therapist.

One disadvantage, in some patients' opinions, is our stipulation that ice be used after each treatment session. We feel that ice should be applied whenever possible, and if this is not readily available at the practice site, the patient should do the program at home. The major disadvantage, in our opinion, is the lack of quantification of the

---

8. Clinical results

164

amount of tensile force being applied to the tendon during the variations in the exercise program. We are in the process of examining this problem right now, but this is not an easy task, since it requires knowledge of the external forces, joint angle, muscle length, distance from line of muscle action to joint center, speed of movement, and so on. Even when all these factors are known, the internal state and tensile strength of the tendon will remain unknown. Until more objective information is available, we feel that using the indicator of moderate pain or discomfort at the end of 30 repetitions is a satisfactory means of ensuring that the tendon is not excessively overloaded.

We should reiterate here that, as with any training program, results will not be seen immediately. This idea is readily understood by most athletes with respect to their own training programs, but may require reinforcement when applied to treatment programs. This is especially true for nonathletic individuals. Ideally, patients should be seen regularly to ensure that the program is correctly followed. Naturally, this is more important during the early stages before the patient becomes familiar with the program.

Conclusions

The eccentric exercise program presented in this book is one that we have used with a great deal of success over the past 4 years. Indeed, it is our standard method of treatment of chronic tendinitis, although sometimes we incorporate other modalities as adjuncts in resistant cases. In this book, we have presented the scientific and clinical background that led to the development of the program and the results of a clinical survey that we conducted. The importance of continual progression, and careful maintenance of discomfort during exercise at a tolerable level, must be borne in mind at all times. Lack of either will result, in most instances, in failure of the program.

8. Clinical results

References

Abbott, B., Bigland, B., Ritchie, J. M. The physiological cost of negative work. *J. Physiol.* 117:380–390, 1952.

Abrahams, M. Mechanical behavior of tendon in vitro. *Med. Biol. Eng.* 5:433–443, 1967.

Adams, A. Effect of exercise upon ligament strength. *Res. Q.* 37:163–167, 1966.

Akeson, W.H., Amiel, D., LaViolette, D. The connective tissue response to immobility: a study of chrondroitin-4 and 6-sulfate and dermatan sulfate changes in periarticular connective tissue of control and immobilized knees of dogs. *Clin. Orthop.* 51:183–197, 1967.

Alexander, R.McN. The mechanics of jumping by a dog (canis familiaris). *J. Zool. (Lond.)* 173:549–573, 1974.

Alexander, R.McN., Bennet-Clarke, H.C. Storage of elastic strain energy in muscle and other tissue. *Nature* 265:114–117, 1977.

Alexander, R.McN., Vernon, A. The mechanics of hopping by kangaroos (Macropodiae). *J. Zool. (Lond.)* 177:265–303, 1975.

Alexander, R.McN., Vernon, A. The dimensions of knee and ankle muscles and the forces they exert. *J. Hum. Mvt. Stud.* 1:115–123, 1975.

Amiel, D., Akeson, W.H., Harwood, F.L., Mechanic, G.L. The effect of immobilization on the types of collagen synthesized in periarticular connective tissue. *Connect. Tissue Res.* 8(1):27–32, 1980.

Amiel, D.S., Woo, S.L.-Y., Harwood, F.L., Akeson, W.H. The effect of immobilization on collagen turnover in connective tissue: a biochemical-biomechanical correlation. *Acta Orthop. Scand.* 53(3):325–332, 1982.

Asmussen, E. Experiments on positive and negative work. In Floyd, W.F., Welford, A.T. (eds.), *Symposium on Fatigue.* London: H.K. Lewis and Co., 1953, p. 77.

Asmussen, E. Storage of elastic energy and mechanical efficiency of human muscle. *Acta Physiol. Scand.* [*Suppl.*] 440:1976.

Bailey, A.J., Robins, S.P., Balian, G. Biological significance of the intermolecular crosslinks of collagen. *Nature* 251:105–109, 1974.

Barbenel, J.C., Evans, J.H., Finlay, J.B. Stress-strain relations for soft connective tissues. In Kenedi, R.M. (ed.), *Perspectives in Biomedical Engineering*. London: Macmillan Co., 1973, p. 165.

Barfred, T. Experimental rupture of the Achilles tendon: comparison of various types of experimental rupture in rats. *Acta Orthop. Scand.* 42:528–543, 1971.

Barnes, G.R.G., Pinder, D.N. In vivo tendon tension and bone strain measurement and correlation. *J. Biomech.* 7(1):35–42, 1974.

Benedict, J.V., Walker, L.B., Harris, E.N. Stress-strain characteristics and tensile strength of unembalmed human tendon. *J. Biomech.* 1:53–63, 1968.

Bernhang, A.M., Dehner, W., Fogarty, C. Tennis elbow: a biomechanical approach. *J. Sports Med.* 2(5):235–260, 1974.

Bigland-Ritchie, B., Woods, J.J. Integrated electromyogram and oxygen uptake during positive and negative work. *J. Physiol. (Lond.)* 260:267–277, 1976.

Binder, M.D. Further evidence that the Golgi tendon organ monitors the activity of a discrete set of motor units within a muscle. *Exp. Brain Res.* 43:186–192, 1981.

Bistevins, R., Awad, E.A. Structure and ultrastructure of mechanoreceptors at the human musculotendinous junction. *Arch. Phys. Med. Rehabil.* 62:74–82, 1981.

Blanton, P.L., Biggs, N.L. Ultimate tensile strength of fetal and adult human tendons. *J. Biomech.* 3:181–189, 1970.

Blazina, M. Jumper's knee. *Orthop. Clin. North Am.* 2:665–678, 1973.

Bonde-Peterson, F., Knuttgen, H.G. Effects of training with eccentric muscle contraction on human muscle metabolites. *Acta Physiol. Scand.* 80:16A–17A, 1970.

Booth, F.W., Gould, E.W. Effects of training and disuse on connective tissue. *Exerc. Sport Sci. Rev.* 3:83–107, 1975.

Bosco, C., Komi, P.V. Potentiation of the mechanical behavior of the human skeletal muscle through pre-stretching. *Acta. Physiol. Scand.* 106:467–472, 1979.

Bosco, C., Komi, P.V., Luhtanen, P., et al. Neuromuscular function and mechanical efficiency of human leg extensor muscles during jumping exercises. *Acta Physiol. Scand.* 114:543–550, 1982.

Bosco, C., Viitasalo, J.T., Komi, P.V., Luhtanen, P. Combined effect of elastic energy and myoelectrical potentiation during stretch-shortening cycle exercise. *Acta Physiol. Scand.* 114:557–565, 1982.

Boyd, H.B., McLeod, A.C. Tennis elbow. *J. Bone Joint Surg.* 55A(6):1183–1187, 1973.

References

Brown, J.H. Dimethyl sulfoxide (DMSO)—a unique therapeutic entity. *Aviat. Space Environ. Med.* 53(1):82–90, 1982.

Brown, T.D., Fu, F.H., Hanley, E.N. Comparative assessment of the early mechanical integrity of repaired tendo Achilles ruptures in the rabbit. *J. Trauma* 21(11):951–957, 1981.

Burry, H.C. Soft tissue injury in sport. *Exerc. Sport Sci. Rev.* 3:275–298, 1975.

Butler, D.L., Grood, E.S., Noyes, F.R., Zernicke, R.F. Biomechanics of ligaments and tendons. *Exerc. Sport Sci. Rev.* 6:125–182, 1978.

Cavagna, G.A. Power output of a previously stretched muscle. *Med. Sport* 6:159–167, 1971.

Cavagna, G., Dusman, B., Margaria, R. Positive work done by a previously stretched muscle. *J. Appl. Physiol.* 24:21–32, 1968.

Cavagna, G.A., Kaneko, M. Mechanical work and efficiency in level walking and running. *J. Physiol.* 168:467–481, 1977.

Cavagna, G.A., Komarek, L., Mazzoleni, S. The mechanics of sprint running. *J. Physiol.* 217:709–721, 1971.

Cavagna, G.A., Margaria, R. Mechanics of walking. *J. Appl. Physiol.* 21(1):271–278, 1966.

Cavagna, G.A., Saibene, F.P., Margaria, R. Mechanical work in running. *J. Appl. Physiol.* 19(2):249–256, 1965.

Cavagna, G.A., Saibene, F.P., Margaria, R. Effect of negative work on the amount of positive work performed by an isolated muscle. *J. Appl. Physiol.* 20(1):157–158, 1965.

Cavagna, G.A., Thys, H., Zamboni, A. The sources of external work in level walking and running. *J. Physiol.* 262:639–657, 1976.

Chvapil, M. *Physiology of Connective Tissue.* London: Butterworth, 1967.

Clancy, W.G. Tendinitis and plantar fasciitis in runners. In D'Ambrosia, R., and Drez, D., Jr. (eds.), *Prevention and Treatment of Running Injuries.* Thorofare, N.J.: Charles B. Slack, 1982, pp. 77–88.

Clancy, W.G., Neidhart, D., Brand, R.L. Achilles tendinitis in runners: a report of five cases. *Am. J. Sports Med.* 4(2):46–56, 1976.

Clayton, M.L., Miles, J.S., Abdulla, M. Experimental investigations of ligamentous healing. *Clin. Orthop.* 61:146–153, 1968.

Comninou, M., Yannas, I.V. Dependence of stress-strain non-linearity of connective tissues on the geometry of the collagen fibers. *J. Biomech.* 9:427, 1976.

Coonrad, R., Hooper, R. Tennis elbow: its course, natural history, conservative and surgical management. *J. Bone Joint Surg.* 55A:1177–1182, 1973.

References

Crago, P.E., Houk, J.C., Rymer, W.Z. Sampling of total muscle force by tendon organs. *J. Neurophysiol.* 47(6):1069–1083, 1982.

Crisp, J.D.C. Properties of tendon and skin. In Fung, Y.C., Perrone, N., Anliker, M. (eds.), *Biomechanics: Its Foundations and Objectives.* Englewood Cliffs, N.J.: Prentice-Hall, 1972, 141–180.

Cummins, E.J., Anson, B.J., Carr, B.W., et al. The structure of the calcaneal tendon (of Achilles) in relation to orthopaedic surgery. *Surg. Gynecol. Obstet.* 83:107–116, 1946.

Cyriax, J.H. The pathology and treatment of tennis elbow. *J. Bone Joint Surg.* 18B:921–940, 1936.

Daniels, L., Worthingham, C. *Muscle Testing: Techniques of Manual Manipulation.* Philadelphia: W.B. Saunders, 1972.

Dougherty, T.F., Berliner, D.L. The effects of hormones on connective tissue cells. In Gould, B.S. (ed.), *Treatise on Collagen,* vol. 2, pt. A. New York: Academic Press, 1968: pp. 367–394.

Dunphy, J.E., Udupa, K.N. Chemical and histochemical sequences in the normal healing of wounds. *N. Engl. J. Med.* 253(20):847–851, 1930.

Dyer, R.F., Enna, C.D. Ultrastructural features of adult human tendon. *Cell Tissue Res.* 168:247–259, 1976.

Elliott, D.H. The biomechanical properties of tendon in relation to muscular strength. *Ann. Phys. Med.* 9:1–7, 1967.

Elliott, D.H. Structure and function of mammalian tendon. *Biol. Rev.* 40:392–421, 1965.

Engin, A.E., Kaleps, I. Active muscle torques about long-bone axes of major human joints. *Aviat. Space Environ. Med.* 51(6):551–555, 1980.

Evans, J.H., Barbenel, J.C. Structure and mechanical properties of tendon related to function. *Equine Vet. J.* 7:1–8, 1975.

Fackleman, G.E. The nature of tendon damage and its repair. *Equine Vet. J.* 5:141–149, 1973.

Farr, J.W. Tennis elbow in aviators. *Aviat. Space Environ. Med.* 53(3):281–282, 1982.

Fox, J.M., Blazina, M.E., Jobe, F.W., et al. Degeneration and rupture of the Achilles tendon. *Clin. Orthop.* 107:221–224, 1975.

Frost, H.M. *An Introduction to Biomechanics.* Springfield, Ill.: Charles C Thomas, 1967, pp. 67–71.

Fung, Y.C.B. Stress-strain history relations of soft tissues in simple elongation. In Fung, Y.C.B. Perrone, N., Anliker, M. (eds.), *Biomechanics. Its Foundations and Objectives.* Englewood Cliffs, N. J.: Prentice-Hall, 1972, pp. 181–208.

References

Fung, Y.C.B. *Biomechanics: Mechanical Properties of Living Tissues.* New York: Springer-Verlag, 1981.

Garfin, S.R., Tipton, C.M., Mubarak, S.J., et al. Role of fascia in maintenance of muscle tension and pressure. *J. Appl. Physiol.* 51:317–320, 1981.

Gay, S., Miller, E. *Collagen in the Physiology and Pathology of Connective Tissue.* New York: Gustav Fischer Verlag, 1978.

Gerber, G., Gerber, G., Altman, K.I. Studies on the metabolism of tissue proteins. I. Turnover of collagen labeled with proline -U-C14 in young rats. *J. Biol. Chem.* 235:2653–2656, 1960.

Gettman, L., Pollock, M. Circuit weight training: a critical review of its physiological benefits. *Phys. Sports Med.* 9(1):44–60, 1981.

Gillman, T. On some aspects of collagen formation in localized repair and in diffuse fibrotic reactions to injury. In Gould, B.S. (ed.), *Treatise on Collagen,* vol. 2 pt. B. New York: Academic Press, 1968, pp. 331–409.

Glick, J.M. Therapeutic agents in musculoskeletal injuries. *J. Sports Med.* 3:136, 1975.

Goldin, B., Block, W.D., Pearson, J.R. Wound healing of tendon. I: Physical, mechanical and metabolic changes. *J. Biomech.* 13:241–256, 1980.

Goldin, B., Block, W.D., Pearson, J.R. Wound healing of tendon. II: A mathematical model. *J. Biomech.* 13:257–264, 1980b.

Gonyea, W.J., Sale, D. Physiology of weight-lifting exercise. *Arch. Phys. Med. Rehabil.* 63:235–237, 1982.

Gould, B.S. Collagen biosynthesis. In Gould, B.S. (ed.), *Treatise on Collagen,* vol. 2, pt. A. New York: Academic Press, 1968a, pp. 139–188.

Gould, B.S. The role of certain vitamins in collagen formation. In Gould, B.S. (ed.), *Treatise on Collagen,* vol. 2, pt. A. New York: Academic Press, 1968b, pp. 323–366.

Gray's Anatomy, 35th Edition, Warwick, R., Williams, P.L. Great Britain: Longman Group Ltd., 1973.

Greene, P.R., McMahon, T.A. Reflex stiffness of man's anti-gravity muscles during kneebends while carrying extra weights. *J. Biomech.* 12:881–891, 1979.

Haggmark, T., Eriksson, E. Hypertrophy of the soleus muscle in man after Achilles tendon rupture. *Am. J. Sports Med.* 7(2):121–126, 1979.

Halpern, A.A., Horowitz, B.G., Nagel, D.A. Tendon ruptures associated with corticosteroid therapy. *West. J. Med.* 127:378–382, 1977.

References

Hanks, B.S., Stephens, N.L. Mechanics and energetics of lengthening of active airway smooth muscle. *Am. J. Physiol.* 241:C42–C46, 1981.

Harkness, R.D. Mechanical properties of collagenous tissues. In Gould, B.S. (ed.), *Treatise on Collagen*, vol. 2, pt. A. New York: Academic Press, 1968, pp. 248–310.

Hatze, H. Forces and duration of impact, and grip tightness during the tennis stroke. *Med. Sci. Sports* 8(2):88–95, 1976.

Haugen, P., Sten-Knudsen, O. The effect of a small stretch on the latency relaxation and the short-range elastic stiffness in isolated frog muscle fibers. *Acta Physiol. Scand.* 112:121–128, 1981.

Hay, J.G. Biomechanical aspects of jumping. *Exerc. Sport Sci. Rev.* 3:135, 1975.

Heikkinen, E., Vuori, I. Effect of physical activity on the connective tissue metabolism in mice. *Scand. J. Clin. Lab. Invest. [Suppl.]* 113:36, 1970.

Hirsch, G. Tensile properties during tendon healing. *Acta Orthop. Scand. Suppl.* 113, 1974.

Holloszy, J.O. Adaptation of skeletal muscle to endurance exercise. *Med. Sci. Sports* 7(3):155–164, 1975.

Holloszy, J.O. Muscle metabolism during exercise. *Arch. Phys. Med. Rehabil.* 63:231–234, 1982.

Holm-Pederson, P. *Studies on Healing Capacity in Young and Old Individuals.* Copenhagen: Munksgaard, 1973.

Holm-Pederson, P., Viidik, A. Maturation of collagen in healing wounds in young and old rats. *Scand. J. Plast. Reconstr. Surg.* 6:16–23, 1972.

Hooley, C.J., McCrum, N.G. The viscoelastic deformation of tendon. *J. Biomech.* 13:521–528, 1980.

Hruza, Z., Hlavackova, V. The characteristics of newly formed collagen during aging. *Gerontologie* 7:221–232, 1963.

Hubley, C.L. An analysis of assumptions underlying vertical jump studies used to examine work augmentation due to pre-stretch. Masters thesis, University of Waterloo, 1981.

Inglis, A.E., Scott, W.N., Sculco, T.P., Patterson, A.H. Ruptures of the tendo-Achilles—an objective assessment of surgical and nonsurgical treatment. *J. Bone Joint Surg.* 58A:990–992, 1976.

Jackson, D.S., Steven, F.S. Some biochemical considerations of connective tissue proteins in disease. In Bittar, E.E. (ed.), *The Biological Basis of Medicine*, vol. 3, chap. 8. New York: Academic Press, 1969.

References

James, S.L., Brubaker, C.E. Biomechanics of running. *Orthop. Clin. North Am.* 4(3):605–615, 1973.

Johnson, B.L., Adamczyk, J.W., Tennoe, K.O., Stromme, S.B. A comparison of concentric and eccentric muscle training. *Med. Sci. Sports* 8(1):35–38, 1976.

Kastelic, J., Baer, E. Deformation in tendon collagen. *Symp. Soc. Exp. Biol.* 34:397–435, 1980.

Kastelic, J., Galeski, A., Baer, E. The multicomposite structure of tendon. *Connect. Tissue Res.* 6:11–23, 1978.

Kastelic, J., Palley, I., Baer, E. A structural mechanical model for tendon crimping. *J. Biomech.* 13:887–893, 1980.

Kear, M., Smith, R.N. A method for recording tendon strain in sheep during locomotion. *Acta Orthop. Scand.* 46:896–900, 1975.

Kennedy, J.C., Baxter-Willis, R. The effects of local steroid injections on tendons: a biochemical and microscopic correlative study. *Am. J. Sports Med.* 4:11–18, 1976.

Ketchum, L.D. Primary tendon healing: a review. *J. Hand Surg.* 2(6):428–435, 1977.

Kiiskinen, A. Physical training and connective tissues in young mice—physical properties of Achilles tendons and long bones. *Growth* 41:123–137, 1977.

Komi, P.V. Measurement of the force-velocity relationship in human muscle under concentric and eccentric contractions. *Med. Sport* 8:224–229, 1973.

Komi, P.V. Neuromuscular performance: factors influencing force and speed production. *Scand. J. Sports Sci.* 1:2–15, 1979.

Komi, P.V., Bosco, C. Utilization of stored elastic energy in leg extensor muscles by men and women. *Med. Sci. Sports* 10(4):261–265, 1978.

Komi, P.V., Bosco, C. Potentiation of the mechanical behavior of the human skeletal muscle through prestretching. *Acta Physiol. Scand.* 106:467–472, 1979.

Komi, P.V., Buskirk, E.R. Effect of eccentric and concentric muscle conditioning on tension and electrical activity of human muscle. *Ergonomics* 15:417–434, 1972.

Komi, P.V., Cavanaugh, P.R. Electromechanical delay in human skeletal muscle. *Med. Sci. Sports* 9:49–54, 1977.

Komi, P.V., Viitasalo, J.T. Changes in motor unit activity and metabolism in human skeletal muscle activity during and after repeated eccentric and concentric contractions. *Acta Physiol. Scand.* 100:246–254, 1977.

References

Kovalev, V.D. Loading—the key to jumping in volleyball. *Sov. Sports Rev.* 16:99–103, 1981.

Krahl, H. Biomechanics of the human patellar tendon. In Landry, F., Orban, W.A.R. (eds.), *Sports Medicine.* Florida: Symposia Specialists, Inc., 1976.

Kvist, H., Kvist, M. The operative treatment of chronic calcaneal paratenonitis. *J. Bone Joint Surg.* 62B(3):353–357, 1980.

Lagergren, C., Lindholm, A. Vascular distribution in the Achilles tendon. *Acta Chir. Scand.* 116:491–495, 1958.

Lea, R.B., Smith, L. Nonsurgical treatment of tendo Achilles rupture. *J. Bone Joint Surg.* :1398–1407, 1972.

Lamb, H. Evaluation of effectiveness of eccentric exercise in treating overuse syndromes, specifically patellar tendinitis. Unpublished material, 1979.

Lamb, H.F., Stanish, W.D., Curwin, S. The relationship of eccentrically produced muscular tension to the etiology of chronic tendinitis. Unpublished material, 1979.

Landi, A.P., Altman, F.P., Pringle, J., Landi, A. Oxidative enzyme metabolism in rabbit intrasynovial flexor tendons. I. Changes in enzyme activities of the tenocytes with age. *J. Surg. Res.* 29(3):276–280, 1980a.

Landi, A.P., Altman, F.P., Pringle, J., Landi, A. Oxidative enzyme metabolism in rabbit intrasynovial flexor tendons. II. Studies of nutritional pathways. *J. Surg. Res.* 29(3):281–286, 1980b.

Landi, A.P., Altman, F.P., Pringle, J., Landi, A. Oxidative enzyme metabolism in rabbit intrasynovial flexor tendons. III. Changes in enzyme activity in hypovascular tendons after physical activity. *J. Surg. Res.* 29(3):287–292, 1980c.

Laros, G.S., Tipton, C.M., Cooper, R.R. Influence of physical activity on ligament insertions in the knees of dogs. *J. Bone Joint Surg.* 53A:275–286, 1971.

Laursen, A.M., Dyhre-Poulsen, P., Djorup, A., Jahnsen, H. Programmed pattern of muscular activity in monkeys landing from a leap. *Acta Physiol. Scand.* 102:492–494, 1978.

Leach, R.E., James, S., Wasilewski, S. Achilles tendinitis. *Am. J. Sports Med.* 9(2):93–98, 1981.

Lindholm, A., Arner, O. Subcutaneous rupture of the Achilles tendon. *Acta Chir. Scand.* [*Suppl.*] 239:1959.

Ljungqvist, R. Subcutaneous partial rupture of the Achilles tendon. *Acta Orthop. Scand.* [*Suppl.*] 239:1959.

References

Ljungqvist, R. Subcutaneous partial rupture of the Achilles tendon. *Acta Orthop. Scand. [Suppl.]* 113:1–86, 1968.

Lloyd, D.W., Buckley, C.P. Deformation of slender filaments with planar crimp: general theory and applications to tendon collagen. *Symp. Soc. Exp. Biol.* 34:471–473, 1980.

Lochner, F.K., Milne, D.W., Mills, E.J., Groom, J.J. In vivo and in vitro measurement of tendon strain in the horse. *Am. J. Vet. Res.* 41:1927–1937, 1980.

Luhtanen, P., Komi, P.V. Force-, power-, and elasticity-velocity relationships in walking, running and jumping. *Eur. J. Appl. Physiol.* 44:279–289, 1980.

Mackie, J.W., Goldin, B., Foss, M.L., Cockrell, J.L. Mechanical properties of rabbit tendons after repeated anti-inflammatory steroid injections. *Med. Sci. Sports* 6:198, 1974.

MacNab, I. Rotator cuff tendinitis. *Ann. R. Coll. Surg. Engl.* 53:271–287, 1973.

Margaria, R. Positive and negative work performances and their efficiencies in human locomotion. *Int. Z. Angew. Physiol. Einschl. Arbeitsphysiol.* 25:339–351, 1968a.

Margaria, R. Capacity and power of the energy processes in muscle activity: their practical relevance in athletics. *Int. Z. Angew. Physiol. Einschl. Arbeitsphysiol.* 25:352–360, 1968b.

Margaria, R. *Biomechanics and Energetics of Muscular Exercise.* Oxford: Clarendon Press, 1976.

Martens, M., Wouters, P., Burssens, A., Mulier, J.C. Patellar tendinitis: pathology and results of treatment. *Acta Orthop. Scand.* 53(3):445–450, 1982.

Mason, M., Allen, H. The rate of healing of tendons. *Ann. Surg.* 113(3):424–459, 1941.

Medlar, R.C., Lyne, E.D. Sinding-Larsen-Johansson disease. *J. Bone Joint Surg.* 60A(8):1113–1116, 1978.

Miskew, D., Pearson, R., Pankovich, A. Mersilene strip suture in repair of disruptions of the quadriceps and patellar tendons. *J. Trauma* 20(10):867–872, 1980.

Molbech, S. On the paradoxical effects of some two-joint muscles. *Acta Morphol. Neerl. Scand.* 6:171–178, 1965.

Morgan, D.L., Proskell, U., Warren, D. Measurements of muscle stiffness and the mechanism of elastic storage of energy in hopping kangaroos. *J. Physiol. (Lond.)* 282:253–261, 1978.

References

Murray, M.P., Guten, G.N., Sepic, S.B., et al. Functions of the triceps surae during gait. Compensatory mechanisms for unilateral loss. *J. Bone Joint Surg.* 60A:473–476, 1978.

Nathan, H., Goldgefter, L., Kobliansky, E., Goldschmidt-Nathan, M., Morein, G. Energy-absorbing capacity of rat tail tendon at various ages. *J. Anat.* 127(3):589–593, 1978.

Nirschl, R.P. The etiology and treatment of tennis elbow. *J. Sports Med.* 2(6):308–319, 1974.

Nirschl, R.P., Pettrone, F.A. Tennis elbow: the surgical treatment of lateral epicondylitis. *J. Bone Joint Surg.* 61A(6):832–839, 1979.

Norrie, R.D. A preliminary report on regenerative healing in the equine tendon. *Am. J. Vet. Res.* 36:1523–1524, 1975.

Noyes, F.R. Functional properties of knee ligaments and alterations induced by immobilization: a correlative biomechanical and histological study in primates. *Clin. Orthop.* 123:210–242, 1977.

Noyes, F.R., Nussbaum, N.S., Torvik, P.J., Cooper, S. Biomechanical and ultrastructural changes in ligaments and tendons after local corticosteroid injections. *J. Bone Joint Surg.* 57A:876, 1975.

Noyes, F.R., Torvik, P.J., Hyde, W.B., DeLucas, J.L. Biomechanics of ligament failure. II. An analysis of immobilization, exercise and reconditioning effects in primates. *J. Bone Joint Surg.* 56A:1406–1418, 1974.

O'Neil, J., Sarkar, K., Uhthoff, H.K. A retrospective study of surgically treated cases of tennis elbow. *Acta Orthop. Belg.* 46(2):189–196, 1980.

Patel, A.N., Razzack, Z.A., Dastur, D.K. Disuse atrophy of human skeletal muscle. *Arch. Neurol.* 20:413–421, 1969.

Peacock, E. The vascular basis for tendon repair. *Surg. Forum* 8:65–86, 1957.

Penrod, D.D., Davy, D.T., Singh, D.P. An optimization approach to tendon force analysis. *J. Biomech.* 7:123–129, 1974.

Perry, J., Antonelli, D., Ford, W. Analysis of knee-joint forces during flexed-knee stance. *J. Bone Joint Surg.* 57A:961, 1975.

Perugia, L., Ippolito, E., Postacchini, F. A new approach to the pathology, clinical features and treatment of stress tendinopathy of the Achilles tendon. *Ital. J. Orthop. Traumatol.* 2:5–21, 1976.

Phelps, D., Sonstegard, D.A., Matthews, L.S. Corticosteroid injection effects on the biomechanical properties of rabbit patellar tendons. *Clin. Orthop.* 100:345–348, 1974.

References

Phillips, C.A., Petrofsky, J.S. The passive elastic force-velocity relationship of cat skeletal muscle: influence upon the maximal contractile element velocity. *J. Biomech.* 14(6):399–403, 1981.

Powers, W.R. Nervous system control of muscular activity. In Knuttgen, H.G. (ed.), *Neuromuscular Mechanisms for Therapeutic and Conditioning Exercise.* Baltimore, Md.: University Park Press, 1976.

Priest, J.D. Tennis elbow: the syndrome and a study of average players. *Minn. Med.* 59:367–371, 1976.

Priest, J.D., Braden, V., Gerberich, S. The elbow and tennis. Part 1: An analysis of players with and without pain. *Physiol. Sport Med.* 8(4):81–91, 1980.

Priest, J.D., Jones, H.H., Tichenor, C.J.C., Nagel, D.A. Arm and elbow changes in expert tennis players. *Minn. Med.* 60:399–404, 1977.

Prockop, D.J., Kivirikko, K.I., Tuderman, L., Guzman, N.A. The biosynthesis of collagen and its disorders. *N. Engl. J. Med.* 301(1):13–23, 1979.

Puddu, G., Ippolito, E., Postacchini, F. A classification of Achilles tendon disease. *Am. J. Sports Med.* 4:145–150, 1976.

Rathbun, J.B., MacNab, I. The microvascular pattern of the rotator cuff. *J. Bone Joint Surg.* 52B:540–553, 1970.

Rasch, P.J., Maniscalco, R., Pierson, W.R., Logan, G.A. Effects of exercise, immobilization and intermittent stretching on strength of knee ligaments of albino rats. *J. Appl. Physiol.* 15:289–290, 1960.

Rigby, B.J. Effect of cyclic extension on the physical properties of tendon collagen and its possible relation to biological ageing of collagen. *Nature* 202:1072–1074, 1964.

Roberts, T.D.M. Standing with a bent knee. *Nature* 230:499–500, 1971.

Roels, J., Martens, M., Mulier, J.C., Burssens, A. Patellar tendinitis (jumper's knee). *Am. J. Sports Med.* 6(6):362–368, 1978.

Schatzker, J., Branemark, P. Intravital observation on the microvascular anatomy and microcirculation of the tendon. *Acta Orthop. Scand. Suppl.* 126:3–23, 1969.

Schubert, M. Collagen and its properties. In Bittar, E.E. (ed.), *The Biological Basis of Medicine,* vol. 3, chap. 7. New York: Academic Press, 1969.

Schubert, M., Hamerman, D. *A Primer on Connective Tissue Biochemistry.* Philadelphia: Lea and Febiger, 1968.

References

Sinex, F.M. The role of collagen in ageing. In Gould, B.S. (ed.), *Treatise on Collagen*, vol. 2, pt. B. New York: Academic Press, 1968, pp. 410–448.

Siwek, C.W., Rao, J. Rupture of the extensor mechanism of the knee joint. *J. Bone Joint Surg.* 63A(6):932–937, 1981.

Skeoch, D. Spontaneous partial subcutaneous ruptures of the tendo Achillis. *Am. J. Sports Med.* 9(1):20–21, 1981.

Slocum, D.B., James, S.L. Biomechanics of running. *JAMA* 205(11):97–104, 1968.

Smart, G.W., Taunton, J.E., Clement, D.B. Achilles tendon disorders in runners—a review. *Med. Sci. Sports Exerc.* 12(4):231–243, 1980.

Smith, A.J. Estimates of muscle and joint forces at the knee and ankle during a jumping activity. *J. Hum. Mvt. Studies* 1:78–86, 1975.

Stanish, W.D., Lamb, H., Curwin, S. The non-surgical treatment of chronic tendinitis employing eccentric training. Unpublished material, 1979.

Sussman, M.D. Aging of connective tissue: physical properties of healing wounds in young and old rats. *Am. J. Physiol.* 224(5):1167–1171, 1973.

Suwara, R. Out of this world. *Young Athl.* 3:59–61, 1979.

Sweetnam, R. Corticosteroid arthropathy and tendon rupture. *J. Bone Joint Surg.* 51B:397–398, 1969.

Tarsney, F. Catastrophic jumper's knee: a case report. *Am. J. Sports Med.* 9(1):60–61, 1981.

Thys, H., Cavagna, G., Margaria, R. The role played by elasticity in an exercise involving movement of small amplitude. *Pfluegers Arch.* 354:281–286, 1975.

Thys, H., Faraggiana, T., Margaria, R. Utilization of muscle elasticity in exercise. *J. Appl. Physiol.* 12(4):491–493, 1972.

Tibone, J., Lombardo, S. Bilateral fractures of the inferior poles of the patellae in a basketball player. *Am. J. Sports Med.* 9(4):215–216, 1981.

Tipton, C.M., James, S.L., Mergner, W. Influence of exercise in strength of medial collateral ligaments of dogs. *Am. J. Physiol.* 218:894–902, 1970.

Tipton, C.M., Matthes, R.D., Martin, R.K. Influence of age and sex on the strength of bone-ligament junctions in the knee joints of rats. *J. Bone Joint Surg.* 60A(2):230–234, 1978.

References

Tipton, C.M., Matthes, R.D., Maynard, J.A., Carey, R.A. The influence of physical activity on ligaments and tendons. *Med. Sci. Sports* 7(3):165–175, 1975.

Tipton, C.M., Matthes, R.D., Sandage, D.S. In situ measurements of junction strength and ligament elongation in rats. *J. Appl. Physiol.* 37:758–761, 1974.

Tipton, C.M., Matthes, R.D., Vailas, A.C., Schnoebelen, C.L. The response of the *Galago senegalenesis* to physical training. *Comp. Biochem. Physiol.* 63A:29–36, 1979.

Tipton, C.M., Schild, R.J., Tomanek, R.J. Influence of physical activity on the strength of knee ligaments in rats. *Am. J. Physiol.* 212:783–787, 1967.

Tipton, C.M., Tchen, T.K., Mergner, W. Influence of immobilization, training, exogenous hormones, and surgical repair on knee ligaments from hypophysectomized rats. *Am. J. Physiol.* 221:1144–1150, 1971.

Uhthoff, H.K., Sarkar, K. A re-appraisal of tennis elbow. *Acta Orthop. Belg.* 46(1):74–82, 1980.

Unverferth, L.J., Olix, M.L. The effect of local steroid injections on tendon. *J. Sports Med.* 1:31, 1973.

Vailas, A.C., Tipton, C.M., Laughlin, H.L., et al. Physical activity and hypophysectomy on the aerobic capacity of ligaments and tendons. *J. Appl. Physiol.* 44:542–546, 1978.

Vailas, A.C., Tipton, C.M., Matthes, R.D., Gort, M. Physical activity and its influence on the repair process of medial collateral ligaments. *Connect. Tissue Res.* 9:25–31, 1981.

van Mamerman, H., Drukker, J. Attachment and composition of skeletal muscles in relation to their function. *J. Biomech.* 12:859–867, 1979.

Viidik, A. Biomechanics and functional adaptation of tendons and joint ligaments. In Evans, F.G. (ed.), *Studies on the Anatomy and Function of Bone and Joints.* Berlin: Springer, 1966, pp. 17–39.

Viidik, A. The effect of training on the tensile strength of isolated rabbit tendons. *Scand. J. Plast. Reconstr. Surg.* 1:141–147, 1967.

Viidik, A. Tensile strength properties of Achilles tendon systems in trained and untrained rabbits. *Acta Orthop. Scand.* 40:261–272, 1969.

Viidik, A. Functional properties of collagenous tissues. *Int. Rev. Connect. Tissue Res.* 6:127–215, 1973.

References

Viidik, A. On the relationship between structure and mechanical function of soft connective tissues. *Anat. Ges.* 72:75–89, 1978.

Viidik, A., Holm-Pederson, P., Rundgren, A. Some observations on the distant collagen response to wound healing in young and old rats. *Scand. J. Plast. Reconstr. Surg.* 6:114–122, 1972.

Wahrenberg, H., Lindbeck, L., Ekholm, J. Dynamic load in the human knee during voluntary active impact to the lower leg. *Scand. J. Rehabil. Med.* 10:93–98, 1978a.

Wahrenberg, H., Lindbeck, L., Ekholm, J. Knee muscular moment, tendon tension, and EMG activity during a vigorous movement in man. *Scand. J. Rehabil. Med.* 10:99–106, 1978b.

Walker, L.B., Harris, E.H., Benedict, J.V. Stress-strain relationships in human plantaris tendon: a preliminary study. *Med. Elect. Biol. Eng.* 2:31–38, 1964.

Webbon, P.M. Equine tendon stress injuries. *Equine Vet. J.* 5:58–64, 1973.

Weissman, A.M. A review of the literature: collagen, its physical characteristics and degradation. *J. Periodontol. Periodontics* 40:53, 1969.

Welsh, R.P., Clodman, J. Clinical survey of Achilles tendinitis in athletes. *Can. Med. Assoc. J.* 122:193–196, 1980.

Welsh, R.P., MacNab, I., Riley, V. Biomechanical studies of rabbit tendon. *Clin. Orthop.* 81:171–177, 1971.

Wilke, D.R. The relation between force and velocity in human muscle. *J. Physiol. (Lond.)* 110:249–280, 1950.

Woessner, J.F. Biological mechanisms of collagen resorption. In Gould, B.S. (ed.), *Treatise on Collagen,* vol. 2, pt. B. New York: Academic Press, 1968, pp. 253–330.

Woo, S.L.-Y., Matthews, J.V., Akeson, W.H., et al. Connective tissue response to immobility: a correlative study of biochemical and biomechanical measurements of normal and immobilized rabbit knees. *Arthritis Rheum.* 18:257–264, 1975.

Wood, G.A. An electrophysiological model of human visual reaction time. *J. Motor Behav.* 9:267–274, 1977.

Wrenn, R.N., Goldner, J.L., Markee, J.L. An experimental study of the effects of cortisone on the healing process and tensile strength of tendons. *J. Bone Joint Surg.* 36A:588–601, 1954.

Zernicke, R.F., Garhammer, J., Jobe, F.W. Human patellar-tendon rupture. *J. Bone Joint Surg.* 59A(2):179–183, 1977.

References

Zuckerman, J., Stull, G.A. Effects of exercise on knee ligament separation force in rats. *J. Appl. Physiol.* 26:716–719, 1969.

Zuckerman, J., Stull, G.A. Ligamentous separation force in rats as influenced by training, detraining, and cage restriction. *Med. Sci. Sports* 5:44–49, 1973.

References

Index

Index

Index

Index

Index

Index